# DEP*

## AND ANXI*        *Y

*How To Overcome Anxiety And Cure For Depression. Overcome Negative Thinking, Panic, Anxiety And Anger. Self Help Guide & Cognitive Behavioral Therapy For Relationships*

by
**DAVID WARD**

derived from various sources. Please consult a licensed professional before attempting any techniques outlined in this book. By reading this document, the reader agrees that under no circumstances is the author responsible for any losses, direct or indirect, which are incurred as a result of the use of information contained within this document, including, but not limited to, — errors, omissions, or inaccuracies.

# TABLE CONTENTS

INTRODUCTION ...................................................... 7

DIFFERENCES BETWEEN NORMAL ANXIETY &
CHRONIC ANXIETY DISORDER ...........................13

The Triggers ....................................................13

Intensity of Symptoms..........................................14

CBT AND DEPRESSION ....................................... 16

How to Use CBT for Depression.............................16

Major Depression ...............................................17

Persistent Depression .......................................... 20

Manic Depression ............................................... 23

Perinatal Depression .......................................... 25

Atypical Depression .............................................27

Situational Depression ........................................ 29

MINDFULNESS AND CBT ................................... 32

Basic Principles.................................................. 32

How Mindfulness is Connected to CBT.................... 33

How Mindfulness Can Help ................................. 34

Mindfulness ..................................................... 35

Relaxed Detective .................................................37

Listening Mindfully ............................................ 39

Life Savers........................................................41

Five Senses ...................................................... 42

Stage Breath ..................................................... 43

HOW TO BENEFIT FROM CBT? ........................... 45

Go to a Professional Therapist ............................. 45

Going to Group Therapy...................................... 48

Self-Help Books ................................................ 48

Types of Cognitive Behavioral Therapy.................... 50

Moral Reconation Therapy................................... 52

Stress Inoculation Training .................................. 52

Mindfulness-Based Cognitive Behavioral Therapy..............53

Unified Protocol...................................................................53

**SELF-ESTEEM** ......................................................**55**

Causes of Low Self-Esteem..................................................55

Self-esteem and Mental Health ......................................... 58

Things You Can Do to Improve Your Self-esteem ..............59

Working .............................................................................. 60

Hobbies .............................................................................. 60

Building Positive Relationships...........................................61

Be Assertive.........................................................................61

Identifying and Challenging Negative Beliefs.................... 64

Using CBT to Help Low Self-esteem .................................. 66

Problem Solving...................................................................67

Mindfulness Training .........................................................67

Systematic Exposure...........................................................67

Cognitive Restructuring...................................................... 68

**HOW TO OVERCOME SOCIAL ANXIETY &**
**COMMUNICATE YOUR FEELINGS** ........................ **69**

Sometimes you just need somebody to talk to. .................. 69

But isn't therapy expensive?.............................................. 70

Tip 1: Understand that your anxiety is natural but..............74

Tip 2: Shift perspective......................................................74

Tip 3: Do breathing exercises. ...........................................75

Tip 4: Realize that uncertainty and risk are part of life. ......75

Tip 5: Techniques For Relieving Social Anxiety...................76

Re-label your feelings from anxiety to excitement ..............76

Focus on the situation or task .............................................77

Accept that things will not always go as planned.................77

**TRANSFORMING ANXIETY INTO YOUR DRIVING**
**FORCE**...................................................................**78**

Channel the adrenaline....................................................... 80

Re-assess your anxiety...............................................81

Anticipate the subtlety of anxiety.............................81

Transforming anxiety into motivation ................... 82

Make your anxiety devoid of adversity.................. 83

The art of centering.................................................. 83

**PROGRESSIVE MUSCLE RELAXATION ................. 85**

Stress and Stress Reaction...................................... 85

The Problem with Stress.......................................... 87

Relation to Muscle Relaxation................................ 88

**COMMON TECHNIQUES FOR PRACTITIONERS AND INDIVIDUALS.......................................................... 93**

Cognitive Restructuring Techniques ..................... 93

The situation: ............................................................ 95

Graded Exposure Assignments ...............................97

Start small:................................................................ 98

Manage your level of avoidance: ........................... 99

Activity Scheduling ................................................ 101

Mindfulness ............................................................. 101

**ANXIETY AND DEPRESSION MANAGEMENT ......105**

Self-Help Tip four: Get Regular Exercises ...........111

Self-Help Tip five: Eat a Healthy Diet................. 112

Self-Help Tip six: Know When to Get Further Help .......... 113

**FORGING INTO THE FUTURE ............................. 115**

**REAL LIFE UTILIZATION ..................................... 127**

**CONCLUSION .......................................................135**

# INTRODUCTION

Most people visualize the idea of saying no to something as being of ill character and mind. This is not the case, however, because saying no is a matter of choice. Before responding to a particular request or feeling, an individual ought to evaluate the stakes and settle on what is best for him or her. This involves staying stern and firm with your decision making no matter how unpleasing or inconvenient it may be to the other party. At the end of the day, we are tied to our actions by the consequences. This means that before deciding on something, one needs utmost contemplation.

As human beings, we go through various challenges in life that make us in one way or another, be anxious. Many people have always turned to counter-anxiety drugs as a method of trying to calm down the nerves of anxiety. People would rather employ supplements as a way of dealing with anxiety rather than facing it head-on. The effect of these drugs is not in the long-term nature but rather a short term. In order for one to counter these stressful times, he or she needs to learn through sheer experience and self-contentment. Ingesting foreign material into your system does not teach you sheer perseverance but is rather a shortcut.

A therapy known as Cognitive-Behavioral Therapy (CBT) is a program that has gained much fame as the counter-measure to anxiety. Here skills are dispensed that aid individual overcomes stressful times. Saying no to anxiety entails the process by which one communicates with his or her inner self in a bid to try and cover up the feeling of anxiety. One needs to own the moment and believe that he or she is bigger than the feeling of being anxious. This is not always a walk in the park since feelings are inborn. Anything can trigger that thought of anxiety, and you may find yourself being overwhelmed with the feeling again.

Anxiety is born by fear and is by this fact that they are intertwined. An individual may be anxious in anticipation of the occurrence of a bad act. So long as the likelihood of the event happening is based on an above-average probability, the feeling of anxiety kicks in. The threat is usually real; it may be physical or emotional. Take for instance you are in the house alone, and you hear the window break, you have inclined to the thought that the threat is real and by the fact that it is using force in entry, it might also be a threat to your physicality.

Emotional kind of threat takes the better part of your conscience. Your psychology is attacked in the sense that you are anxious you will panic at the face of something major in your life. The degree of anxiety can affect your mentality to the extent that you dread engaging in a number of activities because there is the in-born phobia that something ill is going to ensue. Take, for instance, an individual is afraid of flying just because of a previous incident in his or her life. It may be the loss of a loved one or a relative. This kind of phobia is usually particular in the sense that it can make an individual dislike a particular product for no apparent reason. The impact can go ahead to affect every aspect of your life. For instance, an individual with the Phobia for heights would not be favorable when using air transport. This individual will not engage in recreational activities like mountain climbing. This individual may also prefer to live in low tide areas. The individual may further be inclined not to work upstairs.

Invalids with this kind of anxiety disorders are often inclined to draw their fears from a previous event in their lives that might have left severe scars with them. These scars are then triggered by similar events in their lives. Their reaction to these events is usually spontaneous. In order to counter similar spontaneous reactions, a patient can be exposed to events that trigger spontaneous reactions in their conscience and then providing the individual with the skills necessary to overcome these fears.

Learning to say no is one of the skills that an individual can emulate when seeking to eradicate anxiety issues. When in the face of negative emotions as abovementioned, you need not let them go to your head or rather your heart. Use your body as a channel to pour out your emotions. Let them pass through you and then out. You need to be ahead of yourself and even before you encounter those emotions, tell yourself that you are about to go through something that should not define you. In order to do this, you need to learn how to calm yourself down. Have a dialogue with yourself, ask yourself whether you are reacting in the right way, or maybe your reactions are misdirected. You need not necessarily answer these questions, but they tend to boost your inner-self. Believe in yourself that these are one of the many encounters that will be a "by the way" kind of thing.

Stay off thoughts that tend to diminish your stance and ego. In your thoughts, you should always have a solution to your problem rather than creating more problems for yourself. Have an attitude that you will sort everything out. The thought of giving up should be shoved and buried away where your conscience cannot even reach out. Believe that nothing is too much. Have yourself in control. This includes knowing that anxiety has some side effects on your body that include sweating and even shaking. What should keep you going is the thought that it is a stage and that it will wear off and pass. Build a practice of seeing how anxiety enters your body all the way till when it departs. Take yourself out of your body cognitively and take a closer look at that anxiety. This helps you to learn from your experience.

The phobia of doing something might be raising anxiety levels in your body to the extent that you are afraid of engaging in some activities. You need to understand that this is normal and that you need to grow from it instead of avoiding it. Staying away from your fears will only create a major problem when it is your time to take the bull by its horns. When approached by these phobias, one usually exhibits signs of the body trying to fight it. Often an individual will feel restless accompanied by uneasiness in the sense of shaking and not breathing properly. The body takes longer before learning to adapt to such circumstances. The secret lies in changing the way one thinks. The way individual reasons will influence how and what they feel. Changing the way an individual thinks will entail episodes of training. This training will entail re-directing and channeling your thoughts towards something that does not give you a chilly feeling. Changing your school of thought and buying from one that is in favor of your feelings will ensure that anxiety does not keep you from engaging in anything. Learning to live with it and letting it not make sense to you.

Accept that being anxious is nagging but learn to live with that nag. Anxiety usually influences the way our heartbeats, and that is why you will find an individual has an elevated heart rate beat. This leads to abnormal breathing. Abnormal breathing, in turn, leads to breathlessness. In order to counter this feeling, an individual can practice breathing exercise. For instance, breathing in and out repeatedly in lengths. This helps you cope up with your situation. Your mind is your biggest tool when fighting anxiety. What you do not think about will not affect you in any way. Employing a distractor is one way of dealing with anxiety hypes. There are various types of distractors that vary according to different individuals. Different individuals will react in discrepancy to various situations. Peoples' hobbies have always acted as best distractors. When an individual engages in something that his or her body likes doing, the activity will take over the whole body, including the mind since it requires utmost concentration. This way, your mind takes a break from all the emotions. These activities range from going to the gym to even read your favorite storybook. Some people even watch comedies in a bid to laugh their troubles away.

When you say no, it gives you a sense of self-ownership. You tell yourself that you anticipate anything. This helps you to be in control of not how you feel but rather your response to such feelings. In order to stay anxiety-free, one needs to train his or her brain to remain solid rock to the harshest of emotions. This can be achieved through having down a list of things that act as your driving force. This way, you will ensure that you are in full control.

# CHAPTER 1

## DIFFERENCES BETWEEN NORMAL ANXIETY & CHRONIC ANXIETY DISORDER

Considering that anxiety is a biological response that drives a person into taking a certain action, it's accurate to say everyone has experienced anxiety. But then chronic anxiety is something else. You don't experience it once and then move on to other things – no! It's a persistent mental state that enslaves you and it can pop up at the slightest trigger. The following are the differences between normal anxiety and chronic anxiety disorder.

## The Triggers

Normal anxiety comes about when one is worried about a specific thing. For instance, if you have a job interview tomorrow, and then you sleep longer than usual, you'll awaken from bed with anxiety since you fear to be late for your job interview. If you dress up and head out and realize you are not late for your interview you will relax and the anxiety will go away. That kind of anxiety is perfectly normal.

When it comes to chronic anxiety, the worry is constant and irrational. The victim usually has an overactive brain that pores for reasons to alert itself of impending danger. As you may imagine, such a condition makes it hard for the victim to function in a normal way, as their worry tends to cloud their reasoning capacity. A sufferer of chronic anxiety feels as though they are surrounded by this dense fog that hardly lets them through. When you have chronic anxiety you never know what your mind is next going to label as "danger." One moment you could be perfectly fine and the next moment you'd be drowning in negative thoughts. In as much as the victim's brain can mark anything to be a potential hazard, the root cause is usually buried within them, and it's more often than not trauma.

## Intensity of Symptoms

Imagine that you are about to give a speech in front of a crowd of thousands of people. If you are not accustomed to such crowds you might develop anxiety. But when you climb up the stage does it mean that you won't open your mouth and speak? By no means! In other words, normal anxiety at least allows you to act in a reasonably normal way. It isn't obvious that someone has normal anxiety as long as they are competent in whatever exercise they undertake. Someone with normal anxiety can go through their day with relative ease and only give in to worry during their "free" time. For instance, if you have problems with your house help, you might spend the day at work with relative comfort, only to come back home and remember about your problem, which would kick up your anxiety.

For a person with chronic anxiety, they cannot ignore their symptoms in the least. Let's say that someone developed chronic anxiety as a result of their divorce. The divorce was messy and left them a total emotional wreck. They can find the slightest of reasons to recall their trauma and activate anxiety which is supposed to be a protective measure. Something as innocent as coming across a child might remind you of how you fought over your own kids during the divorce. Staring at a member of the opposite sex with certain facial features might remind you of your ex-spouse. The minds of people with chronic anxiety almost never rest. And this causes them to have intense symptoms. The sufferer cannot concentrate on any task when they feel as though a dark cloud of negative energy hangs above their head. They become irritable during the day and at night sleep escapes them. Chronic anxiety has a tendency to crippling the victim so that they have an extremely hard time functioning as normal citizens.

# CHAPTER 2

# CBT AND DEPRESSION

## How to Use CBT for Depression

The term depression has been thrown around so lightly in today's culture that it has now come to mean any feeling of sadness or lethargy. However, depression is much more serious with that, as those who struggle with it already know.

Called the "common cold of mental illnesses" because of how prevalent it is, depression greatly affects an individual's thoughts, emotions and behaviors in a negative manner. Living with depression is like coasting through life, feeling unmotivated to do anything and drowning in self-loathing. Most people who are depressed struggle to even get out of bed in the morning, much less do anything productive with their day. There are over six major kinds of depression, each with different factors causing its arrival.

There are a lot of ways on how to tackle depression. An individual can opt to undergo different types of therapy in order to take their mind off matters and try to heal. Depression is an extremely difficult and complex topic to touch on. With a variety of options to choose from on how to handle this type of psychological problem, one of the most prominent and effective methods used by multiple individuals and therapist all over the world is psychotherapy.

There are different types of psychotherapy but the most used and found to be most helpful for patients is Cognitive Behavioral Therapy (CBT).

Handling the thought pattern, emotions and behavioral aspect of a person, it can allow them to get something greater in life and not dwell on the negative side of everything. CBT is a wide and complex treatment that is known to be helpful in treating a variety of mental illnesses, depression being one of them.

Listed below are some ways on how each individual can make use of Cognitive Behavioral Therapy when faced with different kinds of depression.

## Major Depression

Major Depression is one of the most common types of depression. There are approximately 16.2 million adults suffering from it in the US alone. Also termed as "Major Depressive Disorder", "Unipolar Depression", or "Classic Depression", this kind of depression is characterized by feeling too much grief or gloom, being overly fatigued most of the time, having a hard time sleeping well at night, losing interest in activities that once excite you, not wanting to eat as much as you did before, feeling hopeless or experiencing anxiety, and perhaps contemplating about self-harm or suicide.

However, this type of depression does not typically stem from a person's surrounding or situation. A person could have everything one may dream of and still have depression. Major Depression can last for as long as week or possibly throughout one's entire lifetime. Causing a hindrance between their social and personal life, major depression can keep you from enjoying everything you love about life and isolate yourself from others. Negative thinking patterns may lead you to an unhealthy lifestyle. So how do you overcome it?

Cognitive Behavioral Therapy is one of the most common and effective methods used by therapists to help their clients overcome their depression. Enabling the individual to alter their thought patterns, Cognitive Behavioral Therapy (CBT) faces the problem head on and acknowledges the situation. This does not make any excuses or hide you from the truth, but rather allows you to accept the situation and think of a silver lining for it.

A lot of its success comes from the fact that CBT touches on the most important aspects of a person's life, which are their thoughts, emotions, and behaviors. CBT helps you eliminate your negative thoughts and replace them with more positive ones. As it alters negative thoughts into positive ones, it also impacts the emotions and behavior positively like a domino effect. It also deals with dysfunctional behaviors and changing them for the better.

There are some specific CBT techniques that can help individuals deal with major depression, but most experts would agree that the most suitable technique to apply here would be cognitive restructuring.

Depressed individuals tend to have negative automatic thoughts. Through cognitive restructuring, they can deal with this and replace it with more positive ones that can help them function better, mentally and emotionally. Here's a guide on how to use cognitive restructuring on your own:

- Assess the situation. Find the negative aspect that's upsetting you

- Keep track of your negative emotions. Describe them in your journal and rate the intensity of each emotion.

- Pay attention to all the things you automatically think of whenever you encounter a difficult situation and keep track of how much you believe in each of them

- Examine these thoughts and see if they are realistic or

not

- Generate better and positive thoughts that are realistic and seems more likely to happen when compared to your automatic thoughts.

- Evaluate the process and repeat as much as necessary.

These techniques can be extremely helpful in dealing with a depressive episode on your own. However, it is important to remember that professional help can sometimes be the better option, especially when dealing with depression which can often leave the person feeling unmotivated at all to complete their therapy and hopeless about ever recovering from their mental illness.

Major Depression can be treated with CBT in different healthcare clinics. Individuals have to assess their own state of mind and once things becomes too hard for them to handle, they should talk to other people, like therapists, about their problems. This way, they can live a better life and slowly regain control.

## Persistent Depression

Also known as "dysthymia" or "chronic depression", persistent depression is the most recurrent of all types of depression, typically manifesting in episodes that last as long as 2 years and return throughout an individual's lifetime.

It may not come as powerful as Major Depression but it may still take its own toll on the one that may be experiencing it. The feeling of being sad and hopeless, having second thoughts about yourself, lack of interest, and problem of being happy during joyous occasions may be a sign of this type of depression.

It can also change your perspective on how life works. Symptoms may fade out for a while before coming back as clear and powerful as ever, making it difficult for a person to feel like they have any semblance of control over their lives.

Therapy is one of the many ways in overcoming this particular type of depression. Cognitive Behavioral Therapy (CBT) can be essential in dealing with a long-term depression such as persistent depression. This kind of depression may be an occasional experience for some individuals. There are moments when they seem to be normal and happy, and other times wherein they just can't seem to see the bright side to anything. When dark moments come, it is important to use CBT in handling this situation.

CBT replaces negative thoughts with positive ones and changes the way one may behave around this kind of situation. It can possibly alter your trail of thought and behavior in order for you to see the better things in life. When people with persistent depression make use of CBT, it can be possible for them to get over this long-term illness and go on with their own life happily.

A common CBT technique that can help you get through persistent depression on your own is problem analysis. Also known as "situational analysis", it helps people see the problem objectively and find a positive solution for it. Problem analysis starts with:

- Finding the problem

- Understanding the problem and how it works

- Dividing the situation into smaller parts in order to understand it better

- Finding out what your goal is and what you want to work towards

- Finding positive ways to reach your goal and move on from the problem

Problem analysis can be helpful in treating persistent depression since it can help them overcome the problem in a positive manner. This CBT technique will aid them in triumphing over depression and help them on their way to recovery. It also teaches them how to respond to specific situations that may be complex to handle.

## Manic Depression

Another term for Manic Depression is "Bipolar Disorder". This is composed of different periods called Mania and Hypomania. An individual's moods can be replaced between a state of feeling extreme euphoria and extreme depression. There are different moods for different periods, changing without any sensible reason.

Mania is a severe period that may last for around 7 days which is then followed by Hypomania, a less powerful experience that may still cause an impact onto an individual. There are different symptoms existing to distinguish this illness, most of which are similar to major depression. However, indications of the manic phase may be increased self-confidence, destructive behavior, high energy, less sleep, and a euphoric state.

When tackling something as complex as Manic Depression, CBT can do a great job in handling this illness. Directly impacting one's behavior, Bipolar Disorder can severely impact one's way of life and alter their actions and thought pattern. So, CBT can be a great method to undertake in order to manage one's behavior and positively impact their thoughts to induce better moods and feelings for an individual.

People with Manic Depression can overcome this illness through intensive CBT sessions and talking with other people in order to calm and control their mood swings. This can help them become better and gain better control over their life again. There are a variety of CBT techniques that individuals with bipolar disorder can make use of. One of the most helpful ways in dealing with this particular type of depression is by controlling your cognitive distortions, which you can do by making sure you are not:

- Overgeneralizing - jumping to conclusions because of a single instance (i.e., you miss the shot once and immediately think that you're a bad player and you can't play any sport well)

- Thinking All-or-Nothing – seeing the world in terms of absolutes, meaning people or circumstances are either all good or all bad

- Taking Things Too Personally – believing that everything bad that happens is because of you (i.e. "The teacher was mad at the class because I forgot my homework.")

- Minimizing the Positive – discounting the good things

that happen because you believe they are by luck or something out of your control

- Maximizing the Negative – dwelling on your own failures and frustrations so much that they keep you from being happy

This can kind of cognitive reconstruction can help individuals with manic depression to overcome their depressive episodes as well as controlling their emotions. The process allows individuals to take control of their cognitive process and change their behavior. So, individuals with this type of depression can use this process whenever they feel the need to assess their thoughts and behaviors.

## Perinatal Depression

Perinatal Depression is a depressive disorder known to be experienced by pregnant women during or after their pregnancy. Also called as postpartum depression, hormones produced during pregnancy can generate different mood swings and unusual behavior. This feeling can also be increased because of the difficulties a mother must go through after giving birth, such as lack of sleep and constant care of their newborn child. Symptoms that accompany this illness is the feeling of sadness, regular anxiety, worry regarding your baby's health, difficulty in caring for yourself or your baby, and possibly harming one's self or the baby.

Postpartum depression is extremely risky and dangerous when left untreated. This particular illness can possibly endanger the mother and child's health and well-being.

When dealing with Perinatal Depression, CBT can help mothers see a better outlook on life with new circumstances. This therapy can allow them to deal with their negative and unfavorable thoughts about their new life and replace them with positive ones that will allow them to see the bright side of things. Cognitive Behavioral Therapy will also allow them to adjust and change their behavior that may positively impact the situation they are currently in.

Through CBT, new mothers can see different methods on how to handle their every life and find out better options on how to address various situations favorably. CBT can help these women deal with the way they feel and the way they handle things. CBT is a wide and complex process which involves a lot of different procedures before actually arriving at the conclusion. With this notion, there are actually a lot of different CBT techniques that can help these individuals deal with their thoughts and behaviors better. One notable CBT process that is sure to assist mothers with perinatal depression is the Thought Challenge Exercise. The process starts with this:

- Look at the situation objectively

- Identify the feelings you possess regarding the situation and recognize them

- Challenge your thought patterns and the way you behave by seeing the evidences

- Alter these negative and unfavorable thoughts, emotions and behaviors into better ones by identifying them and looking for better solutions to handle things

Through this process, they can learn how to deal with things better and in a much more positive and realistic manner. This may allow them to avoid any type of potential danger within themselves for their own safety and for the baby. Although this can help them go through different situations on their own, it is still important to get everything treated by a therapist with the proper CBT procedure.

## Atypical Depression

This kind of depression is not a long-term depression. It is actually a subtype of another type of depression, which is Major Depression. However, it regularly comes back whenever life seems to be getting down. Atypical depression goes away whenever good things happen and comes back when they don't. Don't let the name confuse you, the term "Atypical" does not signify its rareness. It actually means it has different symptoms and signs when compared to other types of depression.

This can be challenging to address, considering that you might also seem baffled whether or not you're actually experiencing it. Symptoms that lead to Atypical Depression are increased appetite, insomnia, sleeping for more hours than usual, heaviness in your body, and sensitivity to comments and rejection.

The usage of CBT can be essential in battling this illness. In atypical depression, CBT can be used whenever these phases come back. Through this, individuals can positively change their train of thought and possibly replace negative ideas with better ones. This can give them a positive outlook in life and may allow them to be a better person.

There are various CBT techniques to help individuals go through this depression when they're on their own. A common one is by exercising. It is known to relax muscles, take your mind off of current matters (or from traumatic events), and maybe even allow the individual to practice staying relaxed and calm. There are some types that may help people with atypical depression in exercising to handle their depression. These are:

- Find a specific workout that you actually like

- Identify a specific workout goal that you would like to accomplish (something that is easy and attainable)

- Find exercises that also offers social support

- Make it part of your daily itinerary

- Find something that can be convenient to do

- Even if you feel depressed or out of the mood, do it anyway

In this method, they can also change their behavior towards different situation and learn to act better. When seeking help from professionals, CBT can be very effective. Talking to others about an illness is always brave, but trying to fix it is even braver.

## Situational Depression

Situational Depression may often look like Major Depression;however it is triggered by certain scenarios or situations in life. It is known to be as an adjustment disorder with depressed mood. It may be induced by situations like death of a loved one, a life-threatening event, abusive relationships, or financial issues. These situations may bring about situational depression along with its symptoms such as frequent crying, sadness, anxiety, social withdrawal and over-fatigue.

Situational Depression is becoming depressed over a particular event or scenario that happened, or is happening, in one's life. Through CBT, individuals may see a better way to cope with their situation and focus on a better and more favorable thought pattern. They may change the way they think about life onto a much more positive way and control the way they behave towards the situation.

This type of depression can be extremely hard to handle. When left without treatment, it may also progress into different types of complex and serious mental illnesses that will greatly impact one's lifestyle. There are various CBT techniques to choose from, in order to handle this problem. However, Journaling is known to be quite helpful and calming to do. It lets individuals assess their thoughts, improve their behavior and mood, and also attain a relaxed and calm feature that will essentially help them in the future. Effectively journaling your thoughts for depression can be done by:

- Changing your viewpoint to avoid any biases and to look at the situation objectively

- Writing down all your emotions and the way you feel

about the situation

- Incorporating it into your everyday routine

- Attempt new things

- Stay focused on the positive side and ignore the negative side

- Jot down all the potential triggers for you

- List positive items on a daily basis

CBT can help these individuals achieve a better perspective in life. Simply by assessing your own self and talking to others when you have a chance can give a great impact to you. Talking about your own illness can help you rather than shame you. It is never wrong to be fighting battles of the mind.

# CHAPTER 3

# MINDFULNESS AND CBT

A term you may have heard about in relation to CBT is "Mindfulness." So, what is it? Developed for individuals who suffer from frequent, recurring, and often severe depressions, Mindfulness combines CBT techniques with breathing exercises, meditation, visualization, and other such techniques that can empower one to move past stress and back into more productive modes of thinking.

## Basic Principles

Mindfulness requires you to stop ruminating in the past and worrying about the future. When you are feeling anxious, you know that you can't just stop.[c4] When it comes to Mindfulness, the aim is to help you reduce your momentary anxiety by grounding you in the present moment.

Mindfulness techniques are methods to pull your thoughts from the rumination over past events you can no longer control. Whenever you are thinking of something embarrassing that happened, or maybe an event that you are worried will sneak back up on you, it can keep you from enjoying the moment.

Similarly, if you are always stressed about the future, then you will start to lose yourself in the present moment, and sometimes other people will notice that you are not all there. Thinking about the future doesn't always involve negative thoughts. You may fantasize about a life that's seemingly unachievable, one with fancy houses, money, and more friends and family to provide comfort. Though these thoughts don't necessarily cause anxiety, they can lead to depression when avoiding current problems by fantasizing about a future that may never come.

Mindfulness involves any activity that is going to pull you from these moments and bring you to the present—a time that matters most. These types of fantasies and rumination patterns are forms of dissociation.

Disassociation can be debilitating. You may find yourself so stuck in bed that you can't move. Other times, it can affect your memory.

## How Mindfulness is Connected to CBT

Since CBT is about rewiring your brain, Mindfulness will help give you a way to stop unrealistic fantasies before they get started. Instead of giving into a thought, a Mindfulness technique will help you bring yourself back to the present.

Sometimes one starts to disassociate because they don't want to confront a certain issue. If you are triggered by something or someone, you might mentally remove yourself from the situation and think of something else. This adjustment in thought may help temporarily, but you are still not managing your root issues. You should know how to use CBT Mindfulness techniques to better prepare you for these attempts at disassociation.

## How Mindfulness Can Help

Have you ever sat through a class and thought, "I need to pay attention.I need to focus." Then, an hour later, the class has ended, and you realize you fantasized about what you were going to do over the weekend or maybe pictured yourself on a trip in a tropical area. Instead of paying attention to class, your mind was in a different state, so when you attempt to study, it is more challenging than it would have been if you had paid attention.

Mindfulness will help pull you back to the classroom. Sometimes we know what it takes to pay attention, but we don't always catch ourselves when we start daydreaming. You don't always recognize that you are disassociating until after the fact when you ask yourself where you are or what happened in the past few minutes. When we disassociate too often, negative side effects will emerge including anxiety, confusion, and memory loss.

## Mindfulness

Mindfulness is similar to meditation, but it doesn't have to be practiced in the same way. You can be mindful while standing behind the cash register at work. Mindfulness can be practiced when you are in the middle of a conversation with a friend. You can even be mindful when you are on the couch alone in your house. There are many chances for someone to be mindful, and there are no set rules of when and where you can practice it. It is all up to you and the situation in which you are trying to be mindful.

There are different ways of being mindful, but as you practice more, you should come up with a method of your own. Not everyone is going to find that each of these methods works for them, so make sure you select what is most appropriate for you. These methods can be done when you are sitting on your couch and stressing over something that is out of your control. Or, if you are trying to fall asleep and the depressive thoughts won't stop, be mindful.

Furthermore, when you are at a party and you are worried about how you look or what you are saying to others, be mindful. When you see something that is triggering but you can't leave the situation, be mindful. Basically, whenever you feel like you need more than what is available to you, it is a good idea to practice Mindfulness. It can seem scary and overwhelming, but it is up to you to do your best to keep yourself grounded in reality and not in your invasive, intruding, distorted, and unhealthy thoughts.

Remember when going through these exercises that if your mind happens to drift back to anxious thoughts, don't punish yourself. Just do your best to keep redirecting your mind to the present. It will be challenging at first.[c5]

The more you practice these methods, however, the easier it will be to stay connected to the present and not drift off into the future or stay stuck in the past. You will have a better sense of how to keep thinking about the "now" rather than anything else that is causing you anxiety.

Group Mindfulness is important as well. If you work in a business setting with many other people, then you know that you can sometimes pick up on their stress, causing your own to heighten. If Mindfulness is practiced in groups, it will help everyone's health overall.

Games are a great way to be mindful. Look into free phone games you can play that will help you reduce stress. Whenever you are feeling anxious, you can play the game rather than sit with your anxious thoughts. In a group setting or in an individual sense, puzzles are also great ways to help keep you mindful. You might consider putting one on a table at a party to help keep people distracted when things aren't as active.

Look for ways that you can implement games into your daily activities. Instead of sitting around watching TV after dinner, play a game with your family to keep everyone distracted from depressive thoughts. Or, try doing word searches, sudoku, and crosswords to give you something to do with your hands. Adult coloring books are great as well.

## Relaxed Detective

The following is a good exercise to center yourself and bring you to a calm state of mindfulness. Think of yourself as a detective looking for clues. Absorb the details of your surroundings. Notice color schemes of the area—the grass and the sky or the artwork and the pictures if you happen to be inside. Notice the people around you. Are they tall? Short? Notice hair colors and styles. Taking in all the details around you from the mindset of a detective can help get you centered again. [c6]

### Quote Mantra

Memorize some of your favorite quotes to repeat in your head when you get stressed and need to get to a more productive, balanced state of mind. The Tao I-Ching has some good ones, for instance.

"Sixteen spokes converge on the hub of the wheel, but it is not these spokes that make the wheel useful. Rather, it is the emptiness in the middle. A potter may shape a fine vase, but it is not the vase which is important but the nothing inside which you will fill."

Quotes such as this one can help you to focus and stay centered.

## The Politician Pause

Another role-play includes imagining yourself as a politician. Take your stress and give it a positive spin in your mind as if you are reporting to your constituents instead of beating yourself with it. A little practice can make this technique very useful to you—you can learn to express problems to yourself in a general abstract that helps you focus on the positive.

## Fake Yawn

Have you ever had someone yawn near you and then you find yourself yawning as well? It has happened to us all, and it can be surprisingly useful for a quick and solid dose of

Mindfulness. Make a slow, fake yawn and you can induce this behavior in yourself. This gives you an instant splash of a meditative, relaxed state, and that small dose is sometimes all you need to find your focus.

**Body Scan**

The technique is often assisted, but it can be done alone as well. You should lie on your back, palms held at your sides. The scan begins by focusing on your breathing. Note the rhythm of your breath before focusing on the feeling in your feet, then your legs, and up along your body.

Take note of how it feels to move your toes and the feel of the exercise mat underneath you. Note any aches or pains as you slowly scan your body. Finally, when you've scanned your body in this manner and arrived at your head, finish by taking note of how your scalp feels against the pillow. Open your eyes and you will find yourself mindful and refreshed.

# Listening Mindfully

This exercise is normally done in a group, but with couples who are very close and open with each other (or wish to be), it can be an immensely useful tool for obtaining a meditative state of understanding and mindfulness both with the self and with the other. It begins with sitting close together. Each person speaks, uninterrupted, about one thing that they are stressed about as well as something that they are looking forward to enjoying. When the first finishes, the other speaks about their own single stress and the thing that they are looking forward to enjoying.

The person speaking at the time should focus on their feelings about speaking and what they are saying—how their mind races or how their body feels. They should also focus on the posture of the other during their talk. The listener should focus on how they feel listening and on the speaker's body language. Thus, personal body language can be learned, which is useful enough for the whole exercise, but there is much more to be obtained from this practice.

At the close of the practice, each person describes what it was like for them both to speak and to listen. Some points to consider: How did I feel while talking? While listening? Did my mind wander at all? Did I feel judged or pass judgment?

For couples, a good closing might be for each to repeat what the other person said using their own words. No judgment should be made, but some positive affirmation can be given. Examples of closing remarks are: "Yes, that is close to/exactly what I was wanting to communicate" or "I don't feel that was everything, but we'll keep working at this so that we may both be heard."

Don't expect results overnight, but with this technique, closeness and mindfulness can be improved in the couple structure. Like anything worthwhile, a little work is involved, but you will love the results.

## Life Savers

Take the first roll of candy apart and assign a particular moment of success or happiness to a color in the candy stack. Taste each flavor as you assign it as this is important to achieve the desired effect.

When you are feeling disjointed, tasked, or stressed, take a Life Saver out of your pocket, note the color, and then taste it. Think of the happy moment you've associated with it. Don't overthink it, just taste the flavor and think of your happy place, time, or moment. Savor it, enjoy the candy, and do not let yourself think of the problem until the Life Saver is finished.

Giving yourself a break to think of something positive can help you get your mind back to the logical and positive approach to life. Creating a mental reminder in the candy can help you draw upon that memory in an instant through a physical medium. Plus, the candy is portable.

## Raisin

Less associated to specific feelings, the "raisin" is another popular Mindfulness technique associated with taste that can help you bring your mind to the surface over emotional turmoil or the perils of anxiety. This technique involves taking a raisin and pretending that it is the first time you have ever had one. Note how it feels in your hand and its texture when squeezed between your fingers. How does it smell? Lick it. How does it taste before you bite into it? After? The simple act of slowing down and contemplating all of the stages of enjoying this fruit can have a calming effect on the thoughts, distracting you for a moment and bringing a proper state of mindfulness to your thoughts.

## Five Senses

"Five Senses" is another great technique that requires nothing but your body. For this one, don't get up and grab things, but instead, just identify them in your mind. This method takes you through all five of your senses, the ability to hear, see, touch, smell, and taste. You will also be counting down from five, so there will be less of a chance to be interrupted by more intrusive thoughts.

Start by identifying five things that you can see. These are any five things, and you just have to pick them out with your brain and your eyes. Maybe it is the couch in front of you, or the table that is holding all your stuff.

Next, find four things that you can touch. Maybe it is your own leg, or perhaps the fuzzy blanket wrapped around you. After that, pick out three things that you can hear. Perhaps the wind is knocking against the windows, or maybe there's a dog barking outside.

Now find two things that you can smell. You might not be able to smell anything easily, like a candle or perfume, but maybe the couch you are sitting on has a smell, or perhaps you live above a coffee shop.

Finally, pick out one thing that you can taste. You shouldn't actually taste this item, but there is something in the room you are in that has a flavor, so what is it? What would you be able to identify that item by? Repeat this process as often as you need to keep you grounded in the present moment.

## Stage Breath

This technique is simple to do, and its appeal is that it is quick, portable, and effective. When distressed and needing some quick relief, simply breathe in, counting to three. Hold the breath and count to three. Then exhale, stopping when you reach a count of three. You can alternate the counts for various results, but three will get you started. Try different counts for the steps to see which results are best for you. Some inhale for three, hold for three, and exhale for four. Some do the opposite. Find what works for you. This technique also works in pain management, and practice can make it become automatic when your body and mind find it useful on a subconscious level.

# CHAPTER 4

## HOW TO BENEFIT FROM CBT?

If you are interested in undergoing Cognitive Behavioral Therapy, there are four simple ways of benefiting from it. The mode of therapy a person chooses will depend on what their requirements are, the amount of time they have, and the economic feasibility of it. Read through the following information to determine the best way to acquire Cognitive Behavioral Therapy for yourself.

## Go to a Professional Therapist

The very best way to get therapy is always to go to a qualified professional. Such therapists have taken courses and undergo training to help clients with Cognitive Behavioral Therapy. You can find a good therapist by looking up reviews online or through recommendations from family, friends, or colleagues. You can even reach out to others and ask them about their experience with a particular therapist. Because Cognitive Behavioral Therapy is a very collaborative therapy, it is important that you find a therapist you can trust and that can meet your needs.

After selecting a therapist, you can make appointments and go for the assigned sessions. The therapist will sit with you and ask you questions to understand your issues and then decide on a course of action. If you don't feel comfortable with a therapist in this initial session, you might want to consider finding another one. If not, you can try a couple of more sessions and see if it is working out for you.

The entire course of the Cognitive Behavioral Therapy will usually last anywhere between a few weeks to a few months. The therapist may hold multiple sessions in a single week or only assign one session per week. It will all depend on the client, as well as that particular therapist. The client will be assigned extra homework in between each session, and it is crucial to carry this out if you want the therapy to work. The therapist will only assign a new task after the older one is completed successfully.

The therapist will continually evaluate to make sure the therapy is helping the person get better and improve their way of life. Choosing a therapist means you have to be willing to trust them and establish a strong bond with them.

Opting for Computer Based Therapy

In this digital age, anything can be done online. In computer-based therapy, there is no human therapist involved. It is all done via computer or the Internet. A computer program is designed to interact with the person and provide Cognitive

Behavioral Therapy according to their needs. Computer-based Cognitive Behavioral Therapy is much more cost-effective than a real therapist. This option is usually a go-to for people who cannot afford expensive sessions with professionals. The program is set up to carry out the different phases of Cognitive Behavioral Therapy. It will ask the person relevant questions and then evaluate their condition.

This kind of program helps a lot of people determine if they are really suffering from depression and how severe their condition is. The computer program will advise them on a suitable course of action to get better. You have to understand that the same results cannot be expected from a computer program as a real therapist. However, there is value in this mode and it can really help people who don't have very serious conditions or symptoms.

You can look for the best Cognitive Behavioral Therapy software or websites available in the market. Choose the best one possible and try it out. One positive of this model of Cognitive Behavioral Therapy is that the software will be a one-time investment, in most cases, and allow the person access for as long as needed. Sessions with a real therapist are usually only over a short period of time. This computer-based therapy is considered more sustainable and is getting more popular by the day.

## Going to Group Therapy

Group therapy is another way of undergoing Cognitive Behavioral Therapy. This is also cheaper than attending one on one sessions with a therapist. In group therapy, you will be joining a group of people who suffer from the same issues or condition as you. A lot of people find these group sessions comforting because they see that others face the same problems as they do. They can be more expressive and learn a lot from the experiences of others. They also get support from these people facing similar problems and it can be quite helpful. Listening to others relate their stories helps in connecting to them. You can look for such group sessions being held in many different places. Look them up online or ask a therapist or even a friend for a recommendation.

Group sessions involve sharing stories, advice, and also other group activities. These group activities help the participants learn new things and slowly improve their conditions together. Some groups will even allow you to bring a friend or family member to give you support for a while. Group therapy is often recommended to drug addicts, alcoholics, people with depression or anxiety, and even people with other conditions.

## Self-Help Books

Reading is also another simple way of going through Cognitive

Behavioral Therapy. Some people find it very awkward to talk to therapists or anyone else about their problems. They might not be able to establish the required level of comfort with a therapist. In this case, reading a book can be much better. A good book on Cognitive Behavioral Therapy can be easier to understand and utilize than a bad therapist. Self-help books on Cognitive Behavioral Therapy can easily be ordered online or bought at a bookstore these days. Look through the ratings and recommendations to find the best ones.

Invest in an eBook as well as a hard copy, if you get a good Cognitive Behavioral Therapy book. This way, the book will always be available to you when you need it. A quick online search can easily provide you with both and there are a lot of online stores where you can easily get both together. There are book clubs out there that will allow you to discuss the book you read and also give you a chance to get other opinions on any particular books. You can express your own interpretation of it and learn from other's opinions as well. Look for a book that is like a workbook and helps you learn real skills over time.

These are the multiple different ways in which Cognitive Behavioral Therapy is usually available to anyone who may need it or are just curious about it. It is a good option for any person who wants to reduce stress, anxiety, or alleviate depression in their lives. Finding a suitable model of Cognitive Behavioral Therapy is quite simple and easily available for anyone.

## Types of Cognitive Behavioral Therapy

There are different types of Cognitive Behavioral Therapy that you need to be familiar with. They are as follows:

### BCognitive Behavioral Therapy or Brief Cognitive Behavioral Therapy

BCognitive Behavioral Therapy is a form of Cognitive Behavioral Therapy that deals with therapy with time constraints. This particular therapy will usually require 12 total hours of treatment, and these hours are divided into different sessions. It was developed by David M. Rudd to help soldiers who have suicidal tendencies. This was especially useful since a lot of soldiers deployed overseas seemed to have this problem. Rudd developed BCognitive Behavioral Therapy in a way that would be more effective for them and then implemented this therapy for treatment. The first part of BCognitive Behavioral Therapy is orientation. It will require commitment to the treatment and involve safety planning, crisis response, survival kits, suicidality model, journaling, means restriction, etc. A lot of focus is on worksheets for skill development, coping cards, demonstration, and refinement of skills. The third part of the treatment will be relapse prevention, where skill refinement and skill generalization are a focal point.

## CEBT or Cognitive Emotional Behavioral Therapy

At first, it was developed just to help those who suffer from eating disorders. However, it is now used to treat other issues like PTSD and depression. This therapy involves Dialectical Behavioral Therapy as well as Cognitive Behavioral Therapy. It helps the person understand their emotions better and be more tolerant. CEBT is often used as a pre-treatment for other, more long-term, therapies.

## Cognitive Behavioral Therapy Or Structured Cognitive Behavioral Therapy

The philosophies of this therapy are mostly drawn from CBT. There is a lot of emphasis on the relation of behavior to a person's thoughts, emotions, and beliefs. SCognitive Behavioral Therapy uses Rational Emotive Behavioral Therapy to build on Cognitive Behavioral Therapy, along with some others. This therapy is different from the core Cognitive Behavioral Therapy concept because the format is much more regimented and there is a predetermined, finite process. The input of the client is what adds the personalized element to SCognitive Behavioral Therapy. This therapy was designed to get some specific results and within a specified time. Therapists use SCognitive Behavioral Therapy to treat people who demonstrate addictive behavior. It is also used in criminal psychology for recidivism reduction.

## Moral Reconation Therapy

It was developed with the intent of treating felons who have antisocial personality disorder. This therapy helps them in a way that the risk of them repeating their offenses is significantly reduced. The sessions are usually conducted in groups so that narcissism is not reinforced in the felons. It is usually carried out over six months and the sessions are held only once in a week.

## Stress Inoculation Training

It focuses on the stressors that tend to affect a particular patient. Humanistic training is used in combination with Cognitive as well as Behavioral Therapy. The client will be better able to deal with stressful situations, and anxiety will also reduce. The program is carried out in three phases, and it teaches the person skills that help them deal with stressors in a better way. In the first phase of this therapy, they will be given reading material, undergo psychological testing, and it also involves self-monitoring. The therapist uses the first phase to create a program that is personalized for the patient. In the second phase, conceptualization is continued and skill acquisition is involved. The client will be taught skills that help them to deal with stressors and these skills are then practiced. Problem-solving, better communication, and self-regulation are part of the process. In the third phase, a follow up is done. Role-play, imagery, and other tools are used to teach the client how to use their skills in reaction to different stressors. This complete training will help them to break down stressors and use their skills to deal with them.

## Mindfulness-Based Cognitive Behavioral Therapy

It is focused on addressing any subconscious tendencies and becoming more self-aware with the help of a reflective approach. This therapy is also carried out in three different phases. The client can set some goals, and the therapy will help them achieve these goals through each phase.

## Unified Protocol

This form of Cognitive Behavioral Therapy was developed at Boston University. It was used to treat issues of anxiety and depression in numerous individuals. Unified Protocol involves psycho-education, emotional regulation, cognitive reappraisal, and change of behavior.

These are the different forms of Cognitive Behavioral Therapy that therapists use around the world. Each of these serves their own purpose and are helpful since they are Cognitive Behavioral Therapy itself.

# CHAPTER 5

## SELF-ESTEEM

What is self-esteem? A simple definition would be having confidence in your ability and worth. It is the way you perceive the kind of person you think you are, the negative and positive thing about you, your abilities, and the things you want for your future.

If your self-esteem is healthy, you will believe positive things about yourself. You might experience some hard times during your lifetime but you can handle these times without causing any long term negativity.

If you do have low self-esteem, you will always think negatively about yourself. You are only going to focus on any mistakes or weaknesses that you may have. You might not be able to see that your personality does hold some very good things. If you have any failures or hardships, you will constantly blame yourself.

## Causes of Low Self-Esteem

There isn't any way to find one single thing that causes low self-esteem that will work for everybody. You have believed these things about yourself for a long time and this process can be affected by many things.

Here are some factors that might cause low self-esteem:

- Mental health problems

- Bullying, abuse, or trauma – things like psychological, sexual, or physical abuse, bullying, and trauma could lead to feeling worthless and guilty.

- Loneliness and social isolation – if you haven't had a lot of contact with others or you can't keep a relationship with another person, this could cause you to have a bad self-image.

- Stigma and discrimination – if you have been discriminated against for any reason, this could change how you look at yourself.

- Thinking patterns that are negative – you might develop or learn thinking patterns that reinforce your low self-esteem like creating impossible goals that you won't be able to achieve or constantly comparing yourself to other people.

- Excessive pressure and stress – if you are under a tremendous amount of stress and you find it had to cope; this might cause the feeling of low self-worth.

- Relationships – there might be other people who feed your low self-esteem if they make you feel like you don't have any worth or they are negative about you. You might feel as if you can't live up to other's expectations.

- You feel different – you feel like you are the odd duck or are pressured to fit into what others think is the social norms. These can change how you view yourself.

- Temperament and personality –personality elements like having the tendency to think negatively or making it impossible to relate with others might cause you to have poor self-esteem.

- Life events – if you have had difficult experiences during your adulthood like ending a relationship, illness, the death of a loved one or losing your job could affect your self-esteem especially when you experience many horrible events in a short time span.

- Childhood experiences – negative experiences during childhood like having hard times in school, hard family relationships, and bullying could damage your self-esteem.

## Self-esteem and Mental Health

Having low self-esteem isn't a recognized mental health condition but they are similar.

Having low self-esteem could cause you to develop mental health problems:

- You won't try to do things that aren't familiar to you and you don't even finish a task, like beginning a new art project. This might make it hard for you to have the life that you've always dreamed of. It could cause depression and frustration.

- The thinking patterns that are negative that have been associated to people who suffer from low self-esteem like automatically thinking you are going to fail could happen with time and cause you to develop mental health problems like anxiety or depression.

- If specific situations seem hard due to low self-esteem, you might begin avoiding them and this causes you to become even more socially isolated. All of this could cause you to feel depressed or anxious and could cause mental health problems with time.

- You could develop bad behaviors to help you cope like drinking to excess, taking drugs, and getting into a damaging relationship. This can cause problems and make your life harder and this might cause mental health problems.

Once you have developed mental health problems, this, in turn, could cause low self-esteem:

- Discrimination about your mental health problems could cause you to develop negative opinions about yourself.

- Mental health problems may cause you to withdraw from society if you worry about how others see you. This can make you feel lonely or isolated and could cause low self-esteem. Moreover this problem could influence daily activities like keeping a job or using public transport, and this has a negative impact on how you look at yourself.

- Certain mental health problems like social phobia, depression, and eating disorders involve negative thinking patterns about you.

## Things You Can Do to Improve Your Self-esteem

In order for your self-esteem to improve, you are going to

have to change and challenge all those negative beliefs. This may seem like a daunting task but there are various techniques that could help.

**Do Things You Like to Do**

Doing things you like to do and can do well could help give a boost to your self-esteem and build your confidence. This might be anything like your favorite hobby, caring, working a soup kitchen for the homeless, and working.

# Working

Working a steady job could give you a salary, routine, friendship, and identity. Some people like to work on ambitious targets and they love being in the middle of a busy environment. Others will view their career as just a way to have things they want or they only do volunteer work. It does not matter what you do but it is important that you feel supported and confident in whatever you do. You need to feel a balance between your home life and work-life that is right for you.

# Hobbies

This might be something from painting, singing, dancing, or learning a new language. Think about things that you have a natural ability at doing or something you have wanted to try.

Choose activities that are not too challenging so you will feel that you have achieved something and that will help you build your confidence. You should be able to find some classes or activities at your local library, adult education center, or the internet.

## Building Positive Relationships

Try associating with people who do not always criticize you. These need to be people that you feel comfortable talking to. If you spend more time around people who are supportive and positive you will start seeing yourself in a better light and will start having more confidence.

If you support and care for others, they will give you positive responses. This could give your self-esteem a boost and change the way others see you.

If you suffer from low self-esteem, people who are close to you might encourage your negative opinions and beliefs that you have about yourself. It is imperative that you find these people and stop them from doing this. You need to become more assertive or limit the amount of time you spend with them.

## Be Assertive

When you are assertive, you value others and yourself. You are able to talk to others with respect. It can help you get boundaries set. Try some of these to help you be more assertive:

- Use "I" statements if possible: "When you talk to me like this, I feel..." This lets you tell them what you want to happen without being scared or aggressive.

- Tell others if you need support or more time on tasks that are challenging for you.

- It is okay to say "no" to unreasonable requests.

- If you have been upset, try to express your feelings or wait until you have calmed down to try to explain the way you are feeling.

- Pay attention to body language and the words you are saying. Always be confident and open.

Assertiveness is a hard skill to learn and you might have to practice with a friend or while looking in a mirror. Most adult education centers have assertiveness classes that you can take. There are many books that have practical tips and exercises that you can use. These can be found online or in stores.

**Take Care of Yourself**

Taking Care of yourself physically could make you feel

healthier and happier and might give your self-image a boost. Here are some things you can do:

## Diet

Eating a diet that is well balanced at normal meal times that is full of vegetables and water is going to make you feel happier and healthier. If you can lower or stop drinking alcohol and stay away from illegal drugs and tobacco, it could help boost you are well-being.

## Sleep

Not getting enough sleep could increase negative feelings and this can lower your confidence. It is very important that you get enough sleep.

## Physical activity

Getting exercise can help anyone's sense of well-being and how they view themselves. When you exercise, your body will release endorphins or "feel good" hormones. These hormones can help boost your mood especially if you exercise outside.

Challenge Yourself

You need to set goals for yourself and then work to achieve

them. When you are able to do this, you are going to feel proud and satisfied with yourself. You will feel more positive about yourself because of this.

Be sure your challenge is something that you know you will be able to do. It does not need to be anything spectacular but it needs to mean something to you. You could decide to write to your pen pal or begin going to the gym regularly.

## Identifying and Challenging Negative Beliefs

In order to boost your self-esteem, you need to realize your negative beliefs and how you got them. This process could get painful so you need to take the time and ask for help from a friend or partner. If you begin feeling extremely distressed, it could be better to find a therapist you can talk to.

You can write down some questions and notes to help structure your thoughts:

- Do you have specific negative thoughts regularly?

- Can you think of a certain event or experience that could have caused these feelings?

- When did you begin feeling this way?

- What word could you use to summarize yourself? – "I

am...?"

- What do you think other people think negatively about you?

- What do you think are your failings or weaknesses?

It could be helpful if you kept a thought diary or journal to write down situations or details about how you feel and what you think these underlying beliefs are.

As you are able to identify your beliefs about yourself and where they originated from, you will then be able to change them. This can be done by writing down some evidence that will challenge every belief so you can start to explore other situations.

If you believe that no one likes you, you can begin recording the situation to show different patterns:

- My mother called me today.

- My sister didn't answer the phone when I called but she called me later and told me she was extremely busy at work so this wasn't personal.

- My friend asked me to go to their wedding that will be in the fall.

- I had a pleasant talk with my coworker during the morning break.

These may sound silly, but over time you list will get bigger and you will be able to look back and change any opinions that might have been negative.

## Using CBT to Help Low Self-esteem

Low self-esteem plays huge roles in depression and anxiety. When you don't believe in your abilities, you won't take risks or you only do your work halfway. It is hard to be energetic and courageous to put your best foot forward if you think you won't do well. This type of behavior causes poor performance and your low self-esteem gets reinforced. This vicious cycle will continue.

Using cognitive behavioral therapy for low self-esteem involves a combination of altering bad behavioral patterns and changing the thinking patterns that keep you stuck. When you can learn to alter the main components in ineffective behavior, self-defeating thoughts, and no confidence, you will be able to get rid of the poor self-esteem. By learning to act and think more like a person who is confidents can give you more confidence in your abilities.

Using CBT for low self-esteem might include the following:

## Problem Solving

This helps people take more active roles in solving their problems proactively instead of feeling like the victim or passively letting the unhelpful actions to persist. Problem solving could take on the form of seeking to target factors that might cause poor performance and helping to remedy them.

## Mindfulness Training

This is a skill that was designed to help people get in contact to the present moment and to not be caught up in worries and thoughts. Mindfulness could help you be less hard on yourself and keep you from second-guessing your performance during hard situations and this will help improve your confidence.

## Systematic Exposure

This works with the theory that avoiding situations that you fear will keep you from evaluating whether you are as bad as you think you are. When you expose yourself to these situations that you would normally avoid, you learn that they aren't as bad as you thought and your anxiety will go away. Exposure to boost your self-esteem normally includes a plan to do the activities that you are not confident doing like public speaking, doing it a lot, and using coping techniques to master it better.

## Cognitive Restructuring

This method identifies unhelpful thinking patterns or assumptions that are not true and learning helpful ways of thinking about hard situations. Cognitive restructuring for self-esteem normally targets assumptions about lack of ability or about another person's judgment and can help you think of more helpful, realistic ways to think about things.

# CHAPTER 6

## HOW TO OVERCOME SOCIAL ANXIETY & COMMUNICATE YOUR FEELINGS

Let's face it, nobody likes to open up about their feelings to strangers, but sometimes it is necessary, especially when you're depressed.

## Sometimes you just need somebody to talk to.

Therapy is a very popular way to cope with depression because you can tell your feelings to someone who can give you an unbiased opinion, and doesn't know you personally, so they won't judge you.

It may be challenging at first, but after a few sessions you will get comfortable with your therapist and be able to tell them everything!

If you are not satisfied with your therapist, you can always switch until you find a person that you are most comfortable talking to. For example, many women feel more comfortable talking to another woman of a close age, because it feels like they are having a casual conversation with a friend instead of receiving a therapy treatment.

Say that you are a middle aged man, you may not feel

comfortable talking to a young woman, therefore your therapy sessions will not be effective because you will be hesitant to open up to that therapist. Most people claim that they look for a therapist that is the same sex as they are, but that might not be the case for you. Everybody is different, that is why you shouldn't give up on therapy on your first session if you feel that it's not beneficial. Keep going until you find a practice and a doctor that works for you.

## But isn't therapy expensive?

No, not necessarily! You may be surprised to learn that many insurance companies cover therapy sessions entirely, so you more than likely won't have to pay to see someone. Always call your insurance company to find out if they cover therapy before you go!

Statistical polls show that nearly 1 out of 5 Americans have visited a therapist at some point in their lives. Almost all of these people found their therapy sessions helpful and beneficial in improving their mental health. Why not give it a try? Out of this group of Americans, a large majority of them (over half) suffer from depression.

In addition, if you are feeling sad, overwhelmed, stressed, or annoyed, therapy is a great way to sort out your emotions before you develop depression. In fact, many people find out that they have depression after talking with a therapist. Patients that receive therapeutic treatment often leave their treatment sessions feeling empowered, because psychologists and psychiatrists offer expert advice on how to take charge of their lives and cope with sadness.

When you go to therapy, you might even learn about new strengths and talents that you didn't know you had prior to your visit!

Therapy sessions are always confidential too, so nobody will know what you talked about with your psychiatrist or psychologist. Nobody will even know that you attend therapy unless you tell them. A breach of your security and private information by the therapist is illegal.

Many people aren't sure about the difference between psychiatrist and psychologists, and while these differentiating therapists typically offer the same effectiveness of treatment, there is a large difference between them. The main difference between a psychiatrist and a psychologist is that psychiatrists have doctorate degrees in psychology and are able to prescribe medication for any mental illnesses they may think are present. A psychologist, on the other hand, typically has certificates and licenses in psychology instead of a doctorate degree. Psychologists aren't able to prescribe medications either.

Much like regular medical doctors, many therapists specialize in different aspects of mental processes. For example, there are therapists that specifically specialize in treating and managing depression! A quick Google search will show if any of these specialists are available in your area.

One specific type of therapy that you may consider trying is cognitive therapy. A fairly new alternative method to battling depression, cognitive therapy surrounds the concept that negative thoughts create negative illnesses such as depression.

When you attend cognitive therapy, your mentor will teach you mindful and positive ways to think in order to ensure positive outcomes in your life. This will include not blaming yourself when things go wrong, and not beating yourself up about your faults. Cognitive therapy will change your thought pattern from bleak and hopeless, to optimistic and productive.

The reason for this therapy is that many people with depression have feelings of worthlessness and self-doubt. In order to change your depression, you must first change the way in which you view and think about yourself. From there, your depression will subside and your self-esteem will soar!

In addition to cognitive therapy, you may consider trying marital therapy or group therapy if you feel that your depression may stem from an unsupportive spouse or relative.

That way, you can both (or all) receive treatment to manage your relationship together so that everyone can be happy, productive, and more loving towards one another.

You may also consider trying group therapy if one of more of your relatives suffer from depression as you do. That way, you can both work towards eliminating the cause of your sadness, which may turn out to be the same shared problem. A shared solution would be desirable if both of your depression symptoms are damaging your relationship in a negative way. That way, you can improve your relationship while overcoming your depression. It's a win-win situation for everyone involved!

Contrary to many people's beliefs, going to a therapist does not mean that you are crazy! You just need someone to talk to, everyone does at some point, and therapists are only here to help! You are only crazy if you deny the chance to improve your life and overcome your sadness. The journey to happiness may be difficult, but it will make you a stronger and more resilient person afterwards. If you have a chance to attend therapy sessions, you should take full advantage of it!

The next time you are feeling depressed, you might want to consider receiving a professional opinion, and you might leave your therapy session feeling more inspired! Remember, therapists are always there to help, so don't be shy to reach out to one if you need somebody to talk to. Help is only a scheduled appointment away!

Tips for Dealing with Social Anxiety and Improving Your Self Confidence in Public

If social anxiety is getting in the way of your life outside of work and home, then fear no more! Read this chapter to learn effective ways to conquer your social anxiety.

# Tip 1: Understand that your anxiety is natural but **does not necessarily reflect reality.**

It's okay to be afraid. Fear and anxiety are normal bodily reactions that everyone experiences. Do not beat yourself up just because you have social anxiety. You are not alone in that.

Always keep in mind, however, that your anxieties are just that—anxieties. They aren't real, and you can control or cope with them. You just have to choose not to be controlled by your fears.

## Tip 2: Shift perspective.

Sometimes, all you need to do to get rid of your anxiety for the moment is to shift your perspective. If you think you feel nervous, relax and calmly tell yourself that you are merely excited. Exchange a negative thought or emotion with a positive one and focus on that instead. You should feel better and more capable after you see things from a different point of view.

## Tip 3: Do breathing exercises.

Controlling the way you breathe can positively influence how you feel in certain situations. For example, if you are feeling anxious to speak in front of a crowd of people, it would help if you took deep, steady breaths before facing your audience. By breathing slowly and deeply you are training your body to calm down and focus on the task at hand.

## Tip 4: Realize that uncertainty and risk are part of life.

Sometimes you simply cannot control everything. You must learn to at least tolerate your feelings of uncertainty. You will only truly change and grow if you accept that uncertainties and risks are all part of life, and that not all of these things are bad.

Relax and enjoy life. Face the fact that sometimes, your anxieties are rooted in worries and fears that you constructed for yourself. Let go and dare to be a self-confident individual who embraces life.

## Tip 5: Techniques For Relieving Social Anxiety

Below are the techniques that will help you relieve yourself from social anxiety.

Accept that anxiety is a natural response

It is normal to feel anxious, especially if we are uncertain of the results that we can get by engaging in it. This is also true with other people. Even the person that you think is very outgoing and confident sometimes experience "jitters" whenever they need to interact. However, it is anxiety that enables us to do our best. Because of the "adrenaline rush" brought by anxiety, we are able to function even when faced with situations that cause it.

## Re-label your feelings from anxiety to excitement

Since too much anxiety can influence individuals to acquire negative thoughts, why not associate your feeling with excitement? After all, both produce the same physiological reaction (sweating, shaking, racing heart, etc.). By doing so, your mind will conceive positive thoughts.

Breathe slow and deep

Having too much anxiety can become uncontrollable, especially if physiological reactions start to manifest. You can be naturally calm by taking slow and deep breaths whenever you feel nervous. Not only will it slow down your heartbeat, it will also slow down any reactions associated with this feeling, helping you more relaxed.

## Focus on the situation or task

Anxious individuals tend to focus on the possible negative results and the consequences that will be experienced once it happens. But rather than focus on these things, it would be best if you focus on what you want to do and how will you do it. By thinking too much of the former, you are more prone to committing the mistakes that you don't want to happen.

## Accept that things will not always go as planned

No person can control what will happen. Even with enough practice in dealing with different social situations, you may find people who do not find you as likeable or will approve of you. Just continue interacting with others, as there are other people who will accept and appreciate you.

# CHAPTER 7

# TRANSFORMING ANXIETY INTO YOUR DRIVING FORCE

We feel anxious around various people, things, or even animals. Due to this, our confidence is compromised in a bid to create a balance of emotions in the body. Anxiety and self-confidence are directly related in the sense that an increase in anxiety will lead to a decrease in the other variable and vice versa. Poor self-confidence does not always end up as a success story. When anxiety first dawns on you, accept it learn it, and embrace it in order to prevent it from taking advantage of you again. The lack of self-confidence can be pegged on a number of factors that are not limited to the phobia of being assessed by others. This is often as a result of always looking at yourself in the shoes of others. In order to overcome this condition, one needs to take himself outside the context of a group and visualize themselves as individuals.

Staying conscious and knowing your fears is one way of overcoming this kind of feeling. As long as we are wary of the situations that keep our feet on toes, we can learn to embrace them and in turn, we live a better life that is not full of self-criticism. When self-confidence overpowers anxiety, we tend to be obliged to think on the positive mostly and as a result, anxiety levels drop.

There are a number of practices that might be of key importance when dealing with stress levels.

Know that you have a controlling effect of about forty percent on what you experience.

As human beings, what we experience has a lot of impact in our thinking which in turn affects what we do thus our actions. What we experience either influences us negatively or positively according to how we process our information. In a bid to secure happiness, we are influenced by goals that we set to achieve and the relationships that we are in either consanguinity or affinity.

Your focus should be on events that have a positive effect

When something positive happens, you should take time and acknowledge yourself for that. This has an effect on building self-confidence. It, in turn, helps store the events in the long-term memory.

Fake it until you feel it. You are obviously feeling anxious because your self-confidence has left you deserted and suddenly you feel like you are all alone. This feeling can be eradicated by bringing in face value of what you want to feel. Keep the face value until it becomes part of you. This will involve doing a reality check on yourself and changing a few things on how you operate. For instance, that embraces a posture that is apt, smile, pretend to feel at home.

Moreover, there are a number of ways in which an individual with anxiety disorders may channel the anxiety into a driving force. The issue with people with anxiety disorders is not the feeling itself but rather the response towards the overwhelming adrenaline. There are a number of responses that may be of aid:

## Channel the adrenaline

When one is anxious, the adrenal glands secrete a hormone that is known as adrenaline. Adrenaline is often enhanced by other products such as caffeine. When the body is producing adrenaline, this means that its functioning is at its optimum and that you are able to engage in a number of activities at the same time. Instead of holding back to this kind of energy, one needs to convert it into a helping agent rather than sitting on it.

When it comes to sports, being anxious is the best way to enter a game. Anxiety keeps the players hyped and focused. With all the overwhelming emotions, particularly phobia, research has it that there is some amount of sweetness that comes with one being anxious. Further, the brain processed a lot of information at ago when the anxiety levels are slightly heightened. Adrenaline has its pros and cons. The only way of living through anxiety is by using the pros to your advantage.

## Re-assess your anxiety

Most people have a pre-determined tendency that is directed towards anxiety. People always associate anxiety with negative events that happen in their lives. They tend to believe that when they are feeling anxious, a bad deed usually tends to ensue. This may not be the case. The difference between a feeling of excitement and a feeling of nervousness is almost the same and can be replaced with one for the other. People tend to confuse this fact, and that is why they always relate anxiety to bad deeds. Naturally, our bodies are meant to respond to stressful events through being anxious. When an individual is excited, the focus is often directed to success rather than failures.

## Anticipate the subtlety of anxiety

When engaging various tasks, an individual may feel anxious or excited depending on the past experiences of that particular individual. The best way to overcome such feelings is being in a position to understand and accept anxiety as part of you. Most individuals will be inclined to the thought that artificial counter-measures may be of aid. This may not be the case since they only operate on a short term basis. The more comfortable you will be around anxiety is the only way that you will learn to live with it.

## Transforming anxiety into motivation

In order to transform your anxiety into motivation, you need to find the urge behind looking for a motivating factor. With a little anxiety, just enough to keep an individual on course, this is the urge that you need to find. Whatever the worry maybe, this urge will often act against its forces. You will be thinking of a solution to your problem even before you know it. Anxiety often happens in anticipation of the occurrence of a future event that is directly or indirectly related to you. The right levels of anxiety keep you proper, but when the levels sky-rocket, the demerits fall squarely on you.

Differentiate between productive tension and non-productive tension

Productive tension entails focusing on the events that can be influenced by you. This includes focusing on how to better yourself and move forward. Unproductive tension, on the other hand, adopts a form of wishful thinking since the thoughts of an individual are glued on events that he or she has no control over whatsoever.

For instance, if your tension is focused on a game that you are supposed to play, you will acknowledge your fears and take the requisite steps for instance training in order to make sure that you are up to the task when it falls in your coat. Unproductive thinking, for instance, is when you worry about the feelings of another person. This you have no control over totally.

## Make your anxiety devoid of adversity

The anticipated outcome should not take the better part of you to the extent that you see the worst-case scenarios. Do the math in your head. Evaluate the probabilities. In light of this, be honest to yourself. When you have a calculated risk in mind, you tend to know its severity, and in turn, your anxiety levels will drop.

## The art of centering

Centering entails a practice that enables you to do to carry out a performance strategy prior to the actual one. Centering acts as a method of calming down the mind and making it focus on a particular aim. In order for one to achieve centering, there are a number of steps that need to be followed:

An individual need to select his or her point of concentration. This is often referred to as the focal point. After this has been done, one needs to establish a candid goal. There is usually a desire to achieve that has been covered up by the anxious mind. An individual need to have an already established mindset about where they wish to go and what they wish to achieve. This should be stated in a positive language in order to trigger a positive response. When breathing, make sure that you take various episodes of breathing in and out since this helps to calm your nerves. Tension is what eats up most individuals. Know your pressure points and when to release them. This will help you to relax more. When the body is tensed, you may not be able to achieve optimum functioning.

A person's energy rests specifically at the center of the body. Finding this entre is what will act as your driving force throughout your anxiety expedition. In order to succeed in the goals that you have set, you need to see yourself succeeding. Have the right mindset, one that is embraced by a winner. This will push you towards the desired results. The energy flowing through your body needs to be appropriately channeled. In this feeling of calm, you can now be fully in control of your energy. One should be careful enough to know when to see a therapist. This is because there are some levels of anxiety that are not advisable.

# CHAPTER 8

# PROGRESSIVE MUSCLE RELAXATION

Another important component of CBT involves another mindfulness-related process that helps patients ease their way into their therapies. This is known as Progressive Muscle Relaxation.

In contrast to mindfulness meditation, progressive muscle relaxation works on a different approach. Instead of focusing on breathing and other sensations, the goal of muscle relaxation is to introduce the body into a calm state, allowing for further treatment to ensue.

## Stress and Stress Reaction

One of the biggest triggers of anxiety disorder and depression attacks is, of course, stress. It is almost impossible to proceed with CBT therapy when a patient is under stress. This is because the patient will be out of focus, irate, defensive and even unwilling to participate.

With that being said, it's important to understand what stress is and how it affects the human body in order to appreciate how muscle relaxation complements most CBT techniques.

Primarily, stress is defined as a state of threat to the body, which can be perceived by either the senses or by cognitive recognition.

These threats could be anything that you consider to be detrimental to your well-being. It could be that big presentation that you'll be presenting in a few days. It can also be an assailant that wants to mug you on the way home. It could also be your child's continuing poor performance at school that requires your attention.

Whatever the manner, if you deem it to be something that is a threat to you, it stresses you out. This is where your stress responses come in.

A stress response is your body's way of defending you from this perceived threat. Take note that this is a subconscious reflex and is something that you cannot control once it starts.

It is also important to remember that the body does not distinguish between a physical threat and an intangible one. It will still prepare you to engage the threat the only way it knows how: by fight or flight.

These are the only two ways that your body responds to stress. People differ according to their personality types and the intensity of the threat. For people that take the fight path, the body prepares you to engage the threat in a physical manner, preparing you to fight for your survival.

On the other hand, those who take the flight response are prepared to escape to a safer place.

Regardless of the fight or flight difference, the body responds in the same manner; it prepares you for strenuous physical activity. What happens is that the body temporarily ignores digestion, increases blood flow to the appendages, decreases brain activity and leaves most conscious functions to the subconscious. All of this happens simultaneously the moment you perceive this threat.

On top of that, the body remains in such a state as long as your mind still believes that threat to exist.

## The Problem with Stress

Now, suppose the threat that you perceive is something that cannot be fought or avoided. Suppose your threat is that monthly employee performance evaluation or that report that still hasn't been done. You can't really apply a fight or flight response to these threats.

Now, remember how your body responds to threats, regardless of the nature. Imagine your body preparing to run while you're at the office, brooding over these events. It paints quite the uncomfortable picture.

Now, imagine being in such a defensive state for fifteen minutes. That should be manageable. But what if you're in such a state for a week? How about a month? Imagine the kind of burden it would be to be in a state of danger for that long.

This is what makes stress such a big threat to modern-day individuals. Being in a defensive state all of the time takes a toll on the body and it leads to poor cognitive function. Thus, cognitive fallacies are easier to make. This is one of the reasons why stress is closely related to depression and anxiety disorder.

## Relation to Muscle Relaxation

On this same train of thought, it is important for CBT patients to learn how to alert their bodies that everything is alright and to let go of the stress response. This is where mindfulness meditation and progressive muscle relaxation come in handy.

One of the ways our bodies respond to stress is to tense the muscles. Have you ever noticed that your shoulders tend to go stiff as if you're bracing for something? The body sends out a signal to the muscles to contract. This makes it easier for the body to burst into sudden movement.

Because you can't dart out of most threats, progressive muscle relaxation is done to send a different signal to the body, letting it know that everything is going to be alright.

### *Procedure*

Interestingly, muscle relaxation starts the same way as mindfulness meditation. You begin by finding a small corner in which to exercise. It doesn't have to be a large area. You will be lying down, however. This makes the procedure more applicable when done at home.

Be sure you lie down on a carpeted surface so that you won't injure yourself further as you relax your muscles. You will want to place as little effort on your body as possible for this to work.

The flow of the procedure revolves around creating tension in a muscle group for a fixed amount of time and then releasing it. Once you've released tension from one muscle group, you move to the next. This is done until you've covered all of your body over a short span of time. This act creates a small amount of relief in the area that experienced the tension.

This sensation is similar to the comfort that you feel after holding in the urge to urinate for lack of a restroom. When you finally find a cubicle, the formerly tensed muscles that were holding in your urge get to relax.

When you're now ready to begin, close your eyes and take in a few breaths. This will get you ready for the therapy. As you take your first step, take a deep breath. As you draw in your breath, clench or contract the muscles of your first muscle group.

Keep the muscles clenched for about ten seconds. After inhaling, don't tense or clench the muscles too hard to the point that they hurt. Just make it enough to feel a tightness within the target area.

After holding the muscles in that state for ten seconds, exhale and immediately release the tension from the muscle group. It is important not to do this gradually. The release has to be abrupt to allow the muscles to fully relax.

Once you've finished a certain muscle group, take another deep breath and proceed to tense the next muscle group. The same process takes place, with you holding a tensed state for ten seconds then releasing the state as you exhale.

When you've covered all your target muscle groups, take another deep breath and mentally count backwards from 5 to 1. As you reach one, slowly open your eyes and appreciate the new calm you've achieved.

**The Muscle Groups**

The reason why the process is called progressive muscle relaxation is because you move from one muscle group to the next, allowing each area to fully relax before you proceed.

In order for the process to fully work, it is necessary that you follow a specific order in which you target your various muscle groups. This is because each part complements preparation for the next. Aim to complete this list of muscle groups in this particular order:

1. Clench the hands into a fist

2. Pull your hands backwards towards your forearm

3. Flex your biceps with your hands in a fist

4. Raise your elbows to your ears

5. Wrinkle your forehead

6. Shut your eyes tightly

7. Smile a very wide smile

8. Suck your lips in

9. Make your chin touch your neck

10. Hold a deep breath

11. Arch your back

12. Suck your stomach in

13. Pull your buttocks in

14. Clench your thighs

15. Point your toes downward

Once you've tensed and released all 15 groups in the manners described above, you should already feel a sense of relaxation within your body. Because your muscles are now relaxed, your body is no longer under a state of alert. In this state, it's impossible to be affected by anxiety disorder.

This method has been used by therapists and patients that are self-treating to alleviate their social anxiety disorder attacks and prepare themselves for their next activity.

With practice and mastery, this becomes an easily-accessible tool for those that need immediate relief from their symptoms.

# CHAPTER 9

# COMMON TECHNIQUES FOR PRACTITIONERS AND INDIVIDUALS

First, let's get into the different approaches you may want to explore. They are: Cognitive Restructuring, Graded Exposure, Activity Scheduling, Mindfulness, Successive Approximation, and Skills Training.

## Cognitive Restructuring Techniques

Like a system that involves different elements to create the whole, our mind is the place where emotions, thoughts, and behaviors are generated. If one element in the system is modified, the system as a whole is affected. This principle has a very positive potential for restructuring our minds. Cognitive restructuring just one of the tools directed at aiding a client with changing the way they think about the things that are responsible for negative outlooks and low-functioning behavior. With Cognitive Restructuring techniques, you find ways of producing healthier, more psychologically flexible patterns of thinking.

Put this method of changing our thought pattern is a stress management tool. The aim is to catch our stress-producing thoughts before they feed into the negative feedback loop that consists of our thoughts, feelings, and behavior. Then, we replace the stress-producing with more balanced thoughts that do not distort the overall picture of ourselves.

If we dive deeper into this concept, it involves the precise identification of the actual situation that led you to feel stressed in the first place and actively listen to the thoughts and feelings that arise in that situation. The next step is to analyze those thoughts you have identified as stress-inducing. Ask yourself what is objectively true about them and what's a distortion you've created. As a result, you identify the truer, more balanced thought that is a healthier alternative to the thought you initially reacted to. At first, this can be a complicated and exhausting procedure, but if practiced, if you catch yourself sooner and sooner before the negative thought takes hold over you, it will, with time, become an automatic response to stressful thoughts. In this way, you will determine how you will feel and have the power of the outcome you want. You will experience a new way of thinking.

Here is an example of a common thought many of us have that is not a very productive one. Follow the simple steps provided in this exercise to learn how to restructure your thoughts to more healthy and balanced ones.

## The situation:

You find out on social media that a bunch of your friends went to the same party that you weren't invited to.

The thoughts:

**"I'm not likable. My friends don't like me. They think I'm annoying or boring. I don't have any real friends."**

The feelings:

Lonely, sad, disliked, and anxious.

What is the situation that is making you stressed?

Notice what thoughts are arising in this specific situation

How does it make you feel with this way of thinking?

Fact-check your thoughts just an investigative reporter would do by looking for evidence that supports their claim as well as evidence that contradicts them.

Identify a more realistic, healthy thought:

How will you feel when you replace a negative thought with a more balanced one? Notice how this affects your outlook. Isn't this a way you'd like to be feeling more?

In the example of the party, you weren't invited to when we look at the thoughts arising, such as, **"I'm not likable. I don't have any real friends.**" The evidence that supports these thoughts could be: **"I know myself to get moody now and then."**

Now flip the situation and look at the evidence to the contrary. Then, think of an alternative thought that can lead to a more balanced outlook. This could be something like: I know for a fact that my friends like me and that sometimes they forget to include me in every activity. This doesn't reflect my value as a person.

Think about how what has just occurred in this breakdown of your thought patterns and how you can steer the ship towards a more productive outcome. Notice how you feel and identify the outcome with this exercise. Ultimately, you want to be able to say that you feel happier about the negative situation and that you no longer feel stressed about it.

Take note that this strategy does not involve any amount of denial. One can redirect their thoughts to create a more positive outcome by facing their thoughts head-on and investigating them to determine their credibility. More often than not, our thoughts are distorted by old habits, and when we take the time to notice what's going on, we can deduce the true nature of our thoughts.

# Graded Exposure Assignments

Let's move onto another strategy that you can try in your daily life to combat fear and anxiety. It's known as Exposure Therapy, and it's yet another cognitive behavior therapy that structures a step-by-step approach to thinking about their fears. Now, fears can be anything from phobia say of heights or things. Fear is also an emotion that arises in things that cause us to overwhelm and challenge our self-worth, such as in our professional life or relationships. This emotion, fear, is something that causes people to avoid certain situations. In a way, we are still operating on very evolutionary biology that instructs us to react to danger in a certain way. The only problem with this behavior is the danger we are running away from in today's modern world is rarely an animal that wants to eat you or another person that wants to attack you.

Our fears are more abstract these days, and therefore harder to get a hold of. However, through repeated exposure to the thing that scares us, we can master our fear in a way that allows us to feel safe. This treatment is objectively known to have a 90% success rate among individuals with anxiety disorders, but it can be used in a variety of situations as well.

Here's an exercise you can try to help alleviate debilitating fears. Think about when you learned to ride a bike. You probably started with training wheels or had someone keep your bike upright and give you a gentle push until you found your balance. Then, with repeated attempts, it became easier and easy to find that center of gravity, and soon you didn't need someone to hold the bike for you, and eventually, training wheels came off.

Now, let's apply that to a very common fear many of us face in our daily lives. Social anxiety plagues many individuals and can prevent them from meeting new people and establishing a healthy social life. Have you ever dreaded going to a party or starting a new job because of your fear of socializing with new people? Chances are, this fear has prevented you from seeking certain opportunities or establishing a solid friendship group. I'm sure by now; you see how negative thought patterns turn into avoidance.

Taking the example of social anxiety, this is a series of exercises to help you overcome the thing that's causing you to avoid aspects of your life. You can utilize what's outlined in this book on your own in addition to outside of treatment with a cognitive-behavioral therapist.

## Start small:

Throwing yourself into a situation such as going to a dinner party where you don't know many people is not the best strategy to overcome your social anxiety. Instead, you would be better off slowly building up your exposure to the dreaded situation so that you can develop the ability to cope in social situations, gradually increasing the level of the exposure until you reach the goal of the dinner party. For example, next time you are at a coffee shop or riding in an elevator, push yourself to say hello to someone and ask how their day is going. Small talk is very hard for people with social anxiety, but the more it's practiced, the easier it gets. Then, work your way up to increased social situations until you feel comfortable hosting your dinner party.

## Manage your level of avoidance:

If it's so uncomfortable for you to make small talk with a stranger, it's possible to put yourself out there and do it a way that you can cope with. Changing those habits means being more present in those conversations so that you realize when you're checking out.

### Use your imagination:

Otherwise referred to as Imagine of In Vivo therapy, a useful technique to incorporate into your daily life, is to begin confronting the situations we fear in imagined scenarios. This way, you can strategize ways to make the transition into real-life scenarios easier.

Make a list in order of least feared to most feared:

Create a list of the social situations that plague you every day. Rank them from the easiest to the hardest. For example, going to a house party might be your idea of hell, and would go at the top of the list. Asking for the time might rank lower on your list and, thus, easier to accomplish when you make a plan to expose yourself to these scenarios.

This is just a snapshot of how you can use Cognitive Behavioral Therapy techniques to expose yourself to the situations you fear gradually. Of course, if your fear is severe, it is important to work with a mental health professional.

Try making a hierarchy list of the things that scare you. It doesn't have to be related to the above example. Instead, it could be something more abstract, like a fear of failure or a fear of not doing things perfectly. Jot down some situations in which you feel this emotion. Have you noticed any situations lately you have avoided because they cause a fear response in you? Take the time to write them down and order them from least feared to most feared. Then make a plan to gradually expose yourself to situations that cause you to avoid certain activities.

## Activity Scheduling

Following the list, you've just made of your fear hierarchies, and there is a useful cognitive Therapy Technique that is designed to increase the number of rewarding activities you will need in your life to feel fulfilled and happy.

Now make another list, not of things that scare you (although it could be) of a handful of activities that you know are good for your mental well-being, but you usually avoid. Intellectually, you may know that meditation and exercise are extremely nourishing self-care activities that can enrich your mental state if you want to increase the likelihood that you will regularly do these activities.

Activity scheduling such as penciling in a project you wish to complete or going to yoga once a week is especially helpful if you suffer from procrastination or depression. Not only will you get more done, but you will be nourishing yourself as well as building confidence that you can stick to a plan.

## Mindfulness

A lot of research has been poured into the field of mindfulness and meditation as late. Indeed, the current trends of mindfulness classes and apps are an indication that it's being used for many functions.

Cognitive Behavioral Therapy has been incorporating techniques borrowed from Buddhist practices for some time. As such, mindfulness has exploded into an industry of its own. At the heart of mindfulness is the ability to disrupt obsessive thought patterns and train the mind to redirect its attention to something else, mainly the breath. Neuroscience has concluded that this activity can rewire the brain into changing behavior. Think of the neural pathways in your brain as rivers or canals. The more water is poured into the reservoir, the deeper and more carved into the earth the river becomes. Reversely, if the river or canal dries up, the path of water must feed somewhere else.

This exciting subject represents startling innovations in psychotherapeutic practices. There are a variety of mobile apps you can try with free trials and books that guide you through directed mindfulness exercises and meditations. Also, make sure you utilize the skills you've learned in Activity Scheduling to make it a daily practice and not something you will do when you get around to it.

## Successive Approximation

If you've ever procrastinated doing something, whether it's a dreaded task like a deadline or something you want to do but are scared you'll fail like join a dance class, this is a cognitive behavior therapy technique that will help you deal with putting off tasks. Sometimes, we have difficulty completing a task because it's overwhelming, or sometimes we are unfamiliar with it.

Successive Approximation entails deliberate mastery of simpler tasks that are similar to the more difficult one. Just as you wouldn't drive on a highway before you've practiced driving in a quieter street, Successive Approximation works by rehearsing skills that will make the ultimate task easier. After practicing this technique, the task that seemed too daunting even to attempt now feels more manageable.

Skills Training

Similarly, it's not realistic to take on a goal that one doesn't have the skills to achieve. Again, another common area that many people find difficult is a social situation. Lucky for us, socializing is a skill that we acquire. We're not born with it, and like anything that requires training, this such skill is possible to learn. Here is when you may want to seek out seminars and workshops that deal with skills training.

This could be in the form of a training course offered in your area of working with a Cognitive Behavioral Therapist who can individualize a training program to help you unlearn old habits. In this kind of technique, you may practice role-playing, receive direct instruction, or follow a training plan.

# CHAPTER 10

# ANXIETY AND DEPRESSION MANAGEMENT

Depression often drains one's energy, drive, and hope, thus making it hard to do what one needs to feel better. Though overcoming depression is not easy or quick, it is not impossible. You cannot drive yourself to escape it, but you do have some control—though your depression may be stubbornly persistent and severe. The crucial factor is to start small then build up from there. It takes time so that one can start feeling better, but you can be there if you are willing to make for yourself positive choices every day.

Recovering from depression needs action but actioning when you are depressed is relatively hard. Just to think about the things one should do for them to feel better, such as hanging out with friends or going for a walk can be somehow exhausting. It is the vicious circle of depression recovery i.e. Those things that are most likely to help overcome depression are the most difficult ones to do. However, there is a difference between something that is difficult and something that is impossible. The most important thing when it comes to overcoming depression is to start by having some few small goals and gradually build up from there. Base and rely on whatsoever resources that you have. You might not have too much energy, but you possibly have enough to walk around your house or make a phone call to a loved one. Take things easy, living a day at a time as well as reward yourself for every accomplishment and achievement that you make. The steps might seem so small, but they will quickly tally up. For all the energy that you use in overcoming depression, you will get back much more in return.

Below are some six self-help tips that we believed are essential for you in this journey of coping up and overcoming depression without falling into the trap of a relapse.

Self-Help Tip one: Beat Negative Thinking

Normally, depression puts an undesirable and negative spin on everything one experiences, including the way one sees himself/herself, the circumstances he/she encounters, and his/her expectations for the future. You can never break out of the pessimistic mentality by "just thinking positive." Wishful thinking and happy thoughts will not cut it. The trick needed in this case is to substitute negative thoughts and opinions with more balanced feelings and thoughts. Try thinking outside yourself. Ask yourself whether you would say what you are thinking regarding yourself to others. If not, then stop being hard on yourself. Ponder on less punitive statements that give more realistic descriptions.

Stop perceiving yourself to be perfect and allow yourself to fall short of perfection. most depressed individuals are perfectionists, regarding and holding themselves to terribly high standards and they end up beating themselves up whenever they fail to meet their set standards. Combat this origin of self-imposed anxiety by trying to challenge your negative thoughts. Socialize with positive-minded people. Take note of how positive-minded people deal with their challenges, even if they are minor ones, like not finding a parking space. Then think of how you would have reacted if you were in the same situation. Even if you will pretend, try adopting their optimism as well as persistence when facing difficulty.

You may as well have a "negative thought log." Each time you experience some negative thought, write it down in a notebook and what stimulated /triggered it. Create time to review your log when in good moods. Then consider if the negative thoughts or negativity was truly necessary. Ask yourself if there is any other way to perceive the situation. Always remember to substitute negative thoughts and opinions with more balanced feelings and thoughts. In this manner, you will find it easy overcoming depression as well as coping up.

Self-Help Tip two: Get Support

Getting proper support that you need plays a huge role in "lifting the fog" of anxiety and depression and taking it away from you. It can be very difficult to maintain perceptions and sustain the required energy to beat depression on your own, but again the depression's nature makes it somehow difficult to stretch out for help from others. Nevertheless, loneliness and isolation worsen depression, hence maintaining those close relationships as well as social activities are very important. The thought of even stretching out to very close family members can seem to be devastating. One may feel guilty, ashamed, or even too exhausted to talk. When having such thoughts always keep in mind that that is the depression talking to you. Reaching out to others is not an indication to show one's weakness and it will not mean that you are a burden to others. Remember that your loved ones care so much about you and would wish to help. Keep in mind that it is never late for one to build new healthy friendships and improve their support network.

Turn to your family members and trusted friends. Share with them what you are going through face to face talk if possible. The individuals you talk to do not have to sort you out immediately; they only need to be great listeners. Ask for support and help that you need. You might have withdrawn from your most cherished relationships, but be rest assured they may get you through the tough times. Try keeping up with social events even if you do not feel like it. Mostly when one is depressed, it always feels more comfortable retreating into their shell, but being around may make them feel less depressed. you may register and join a depression support group. Being with other people trying to battle depression can help in reducing one's sense of isolation. In such a group there is room for sharing personal experiences hence there is a higher likelihood of encouraging each other and giving and receiving advice on how to cope.

**Self-Help Tip three: Take Care of Yourself** To overcome depression, we ought to take good care of ourselves. This entails adopting healthy habits, having a healthy lifestyle, scheduling fun events into our day, learning to overcome stress, and setting boundaries on what one can do. Aim for at least 8hours of sleep every day. Depression stereotypically involves sleeping disorders. Whether one sleeps too much or too little, his or her mood suffers. Formulate a better sleeping schedule by practicing healthy sleep habits.

Ensure that every day you do expose yourself to some little sunlight. Not having enough sunlight or lack of it can make worsen one's depression. Get enough of it as much as possible. Take a random short walk outdoors, enjoy an outdoor meal, relax on a park bench, sit out in the garden, or even take your coffee outside. Aiming for at least fifteen minutes of sunlight in a day boosts one's mood. If you are living somewhere with very little winter sunshine, you can use a light therapy box. Always try to keep stress in check. Stress does not only worsen and prolong depression, but it triggers it. Always know and understand all the things that stress you out in your life. This might include unsupportive relationships, health problems, or work overload. Once you have identified your stressors, create a plan to minimize their impact or avoid them.

**Continually practice the so far learned relaxation techniques.** Doing the relaxation practice daily can help in relieving symptoms of depression, reducing stress, and boosting feelings of joy as well as our well-being. Try out yoga, progressive muscle relaxation, deep breathing, or meditation.

**Care for a pet.** Although nothing can in any way replace the human connection, our pets can bring companionship and joy into our lives and help us feel less isolated. Hence, taking care of a pet can as well get you back to yourself and give you some sense and feeling of being needed—a powerful antidote to depression.

**Do the things you (used to) enjoy.** While you cannot force yourself onto having fun or experiencing pleasure, you can always choose to do the things that you used to enjoy. Try out a sport or former hobby you used to love most. Paint the town red with friends. Creatively express yourself through art, music, or writing. Take a tour to a museum, the ballpark, or the mountains. Push yourself into doing things, even if you do not feel like it. You will be astonished at how you will feel, much better, once you are out in the world. Though your depression might not lift instantly, you will slowly feel more energetic and cheerful as you create time for the fun activities.

## Self-Help Tip four: Get Regular Exercises

When one is depressed, exercising might be the last thing that he/she would feel like doing. Exercising is a useful and powerful tool for overcoming depression. Research indicates that regular exercises can be as efficient as antidepressant medication at lowering feelings of fatigue and increasing one's energy levels.

Scientists have not found out exactly the reason behind exercise being such a powerful antidepressant, nevertheless evidence shows that physical activity stimulates the growth of new cells in the brain, relieves muscle tension, increases mood-enhancing endorphins and neurotransmitters, and reduces stress. All these are things that have a positive impact on depression. Aim at doing exercise for at least 30 minutes per day to get the most benefits. Though you can start small by doing activities as short as 10minutes as it will have a positive impact on your mood. Below are a few easy steps to get you moving:

- Climb up through the stairs rather than using an elevator

- Walk around the house while making a phone call

- Pair up/get an exercise partner

- In the parking lot, park your car at the farthest spot.

Keep in mind to always incorporate walks and other forms of exercise and activities into your daily program/routine. The most important clue at this point is that you pick an activity or event that you enjoy most so that you are likelier to keep up with it.

## Self-Help Tip five: Eat a Healthy Diet

What one eats directly impacts the way he or she feels. Aim at taking a balanced diet that is made up of low-fat proteins, fruits, vegetables, and complex carbohydrates. Lessen your consumption of foods that may negatively affect your mood or brain, such as alcohol, caffeine, saturated fats, and foods that have high chemical preservatives level or hormones.

Do not skip your meals. Aim at eating something at least after every 3 to 4 hours as going for a long period between your meals might make you feel tired and irritable.

Minimize refined carbs and sugar. You may desire or have a craving for baked goods, sugary snacks, or comfort foods like French fries or pasta, but these foods quickly bring about lowering energy levels and crash in one's mood.

Concentrate on complex carbohydrates. Increase your intake on foods such as whole-wheat pasta, baked potatoes, whole-grain breads, and oatmeal as they can enhance serotonin levels without causing a crash. Increase your vitamins intake, eat more leafy greens, citrus fruit, eggs, chicken, and beans. Try taking super-foods that are rich in nutrients for boosting mood, like spinach, brown rice, and bananas.

Omega-3 fatty acids can as well play a vital role in steadying and stabilizing one's mood. Some of the best sources are fatty fish, for instance, salmon, mackerel, anchovies, sardines, and herring. When preparing fish, you would rather bake or grill rather than fry them.

## Self-Help Tip six: Know When to Get Further Help

If your depression gets worse and worse, do not hesitate to look out for assistance from professionals. Needing additional help does not mean that you are weak. At times the negative thoughts in depression might make you feel like you are a lost cause, nevertheless, the good news is that depression is treatable, and you will feel better!

# CHAPTER 11

## FORGING INTO THE FUTURE

So far, we have learned anxiety and depression are conditions that are regular and painful. The feelings can range from a normal feeling down that can last for several weeks to a severe condition that might need treatment at a hospital. In the previous chapters, we have seen the importance of CBT as a proven scientific treatment in fighting the two conditions. CBT works with or without antidepressant medicines and has been proven to lessen relapse rates.

A crucial first step in helping you deal with depression is getting to know what thoughts are running through your head and to get more familiar with how you react to problematic situations. Many of us are locked into automatic, negative paths. Something happens, and then the thoughts, feelings, and behaviors cascade over one another inevitably.

Careful self-analysis is critical to be able to pause this process and analyze what is going on. Using the four factors we discussed in the previous chapter, we can dissect our automatic responses and develop strategies to address our problems.

People who have depression often have what is known as

cognitive triad. This is the set of three negative views that characterize depression: negative views about yourself, negative views about the world, and negative views about the future.

It is useful to look for any of these negative thought patterns in your life. The first part of the cognitive triad, negative views about yourself, is somewhat easy to recognize. These are the automatic thoughts that include the personal pronouns I, me, or my. You might find yourself saying things like this:

- I am a bad person.

- Nobody likes me.

- I am terrible at my job.

As an exercise, take some time to write down the thoughts you repeatedly have that are negative about yourself. What is the way that you beat yourself up? How do you speak to yourself when a mistake happens? These negative statements are global and seem to come automatically. Do not take time to evaluate whether or not the statements are true. Simply write them down.

The second element of the cognitive triad is views that are related to the world at large. These are sometimes more difficult to spot because many people mistakenly think their negative views are accurate descriptions of the world. Many people with thought disturbances have a vague sense that it is the rest of the world that is disturbed, and only they see things accurately.

A good clue that it is a negative outlook as opposed to an accurate description of the world is that it is absolute: If you think something never works out or is always bad, you probably are overstating the case.

Either way, take some time to write down the negative thoughts you have about the world. Do not evaluate whether or not the statements are true; at this point, look for thoughts which are negative and directed outward. Some examples include:

- All men are jerks.

- The powerful are corrupt.

- Life is unfair.

The last part of the negative cognitive triad is the negative thoughts you have about the future. You might say to yourself:

- My life will get worse.

- Nothing will work out.

- The world is going to destroy itself.

These thoughts are predictions about how things are going to turn out, and they are generally negative. Without stopping to determine whether or not they are true, write down all the thoughts you have about the future that are negative. Do you focus on the fact things will be bad? Are you continually predicting negative results for things you might try?

Look at your lists. To what extent are you generally negative? In what category are your thoughts the most negative? It is crucial that you have a good sense of how your negative thoughts manifest and where you should focus your time.

Many people come to therapy with the general knowledge that they are gloomy, worried, or cynical. On the other hand, your thoughts feel true and accurate. You aren't a pessimist. You might think you are a realist. Evaluating all your negative thoughts as a collective is one way to realize there is a general pattern of negative thoughts.

The act of thinking about your thoughts is a skill in itself, and it needs to be developed. Sometimes it will be difficult for people to establish the ability to analyze their thoughts.

Take one of the negative thoughts you wrote about in the previous section and think of a situation where that negative thought arose. Did you find yourself thinking that nothing will turn out well or that your future was doomed? Describe that situation to yourself. It is often helpful to journal about it, describing what happened, how you felt, and what you did about it.

What effect did the negative thought have? Did it change your behavior in any way? Could you imagine your behavior changing if you had a different thought?

Make a worksheet with five columns: situation, feelings, physical reactions, behaviors, and thoughts.

With the situation you are thinking of, fill out each column. In the situation category, write down what happened who was involved, where it happened, and when it happened. In the feelings column, write down what you felt and rank the intensity of that emotion from 1 to 10. In the physical reactions column, write down how your body reacted and rank that from 1 to 10. In the behaviors column, write down the actions you did. Finally, in the thoughts column, write down the thoughts you had in that situation.

Analyze what the relationship between these columns is and how they interacted with each other. As you go through your life, develop the habit of viewing things from the outside and analyze them in this way.

It might be helpful to fill out this form every day. Make a point to spend time analyzing your situations and behavior so that you develop an awareness of patterns.

Every person has specific types of situations that set their automatic negative paths in motion. You have triggers—things that spur you on into the thoughts, feelings, and behaviors that lead you to change. To address your problems, you have to know what type of situations are difficult for you and trigger your negative patterns.

Sometimes you will already be aware of your triggers. For other people, it is difficult to identify the specific situations that provoke problematic emotions. You might think that you are always sad or always drink too much and be unable to identify specific situations that become problems.

A helpful first step can be to monitor problematic feelings or behaviors. You can check and see if there are some situations where the feelings are worse or the behaviors more problematic. Imagine someone who thinks she is always angry. At first, this person might think they are angry all the time. But if she carefully monitored her feelings and determined when they were the strongest, she will begin to see patterns. Perhaps, in this particular case, she gets most angry at her teenage daughter when she doesn't do her homework or breaks curfew. She might find that her anger toward her daughter was overflowing into the rest of her life.

You can use a simple monitoring worksheet like the one below. When you use it, note what situations are the most difficult and rate your feelings from 1 to 10. When you do that, you will often start to see patterns. Imagine Richard, who feels like he is unhappy at his new school all the time. If he filled out the worksheet, it might look something like this.

When Richard looks at the worksheet, all filled out, he discovers he was unhappy in social situations. He was not listing unhappiness when he was in class or answering questions. He was only unhappy when he felt like he was excluded socially. It helped him realize that academically, school was going well. Maybe he was in band and didn't feel unhappy in band. That could be going well. The problem was when he felt socially rejected.

Situations can involve interpersonal events, solitary things, or even things that are imagined. They can be memories, partial images, or mental pictures to which you are responding. They are often locked into certain times of day, so make sure to ask yourself questions about contextual aspects of the situation.

As you are identifying situations, ask yourself the w questions. What happened? Who was involved? Where did it happen? When did it happen? It is in some ways similar to being a journalist, figuring out the facts of the matter. You need to have a sense of what events caused the negative feelings or behaviors you are targeting.

Sometimes, if you are struggling to figure out what is important about a particular situation, describe the situation in vivid detail. Events exist in multiple senses, including sounds, smells, and touch. When you use multiple sensations, you can help yourself visualize the space you occupied and identify the sights, sounds, and sensations to help yourself trigger your memory. If the situation involved another person, you could ask a trusted confidence to role play the situation with you. They can take the place of the other person, and then you can analyze the situation again.

One common thing that happens is that the situation that causes negative feelings and thoughts is not just one discrete situation or a single moment. Situations that trigger us can evolve. A dispute with a friend can start as a fairly minor insult or hurt and then quickly escalate into mutual insults before you leave hurt and wounded. Your thoughts and feelings will likely evolve throughout the entire interaction. In those cases, it is useful to break the set of events down into specific moments with various stages of the interaction.

Always be as specific and concrete as possible when describing these situations to yourself. When you identify trigger situations in vague terms, you won't get a full sense of what happened. Instead of saying, "My wife does not respect my work," it would be better to say, "My wife told me she thought her work was more important than mine."

When you get more specific and concrete, you move forward in the process of describing the world without interpretation. Sometimes our thoughts color what our memories are. In the previous example, your wife tells you she thought her work was more important. But what if she had said that she does not want to miss a work event for her company to attend a work event for yours? It is possible to remember this interaction as her thinking her work is more important. But on closer analysis of that thought, it is not justified by the situation. Her being unwilling to prioritize your work over hers does not mean she thinks your work is unimportant.

One way to think of this is that the facts of a situation are different than the meaning of a situation. The goal is to separate the facts from the thoughts and feelings about the situation. An example might be that you might describe your child as being rude to her teacher. Rude is an adjective and describes what you think about your child's actions, but it does not describe what your child did. What was the action?

Do not record situations with your thoughts and feelings embedded in them. Instead of thinking, "I was so angry at my mother when she was late," separate those two elements. Your mother was late, and you were angry. The event happened without the feelings, and then the feelings happened.

Sometimes it is difficult to identify your feelings. Feelings are one-word descriptions of emotions. Sometimes we might think we are feeling angry, but on closer analysis, we are anxious or scared.

It can be helpful to look at a list of feelings when you are troubled and see if any of them resonate.

If you find yourself struggling to identify how you feel, look at this list and write down which ones resonate. Once you start to pay attention to your feelings, it will become more comfortable and easier to label them. Some people have never asked themselves the question, What am I feeling?

Pay attention to when you are physically tense or upset and label your feelings at that moment.

Sometimes it is difficult to identify our feelings because we tend to identify thoughts as feelings. We might say, "I feel stupid," but what you mean is, "I think I am stupid" or "I feel upset." Thoughts are closely connected to feelings, but we need to learn to separate them.

After you are good at identifying your feelings, the next

agenda item is identifying your behaviors. Ask yourself, "What did you do?" You are looking for actions that avoid the situation, are impulsive, or are likely to make the situation worse. Sometimes we minimize our behavior, but slowing down and carefully analyzing what you did is important. You might describe what you did after getting angry at a friend as "letting off some steam," but when you face the facts, what you did was punch a wall and break your hand.

Sometimes we describe our behaviors as "giving up" or "freaking out," but be more specific when you describe your behavior.

The intermediate element between the event and the feelings and behaviors is the thoughts. Remember our CBT model. Events happen in the world, we have thoughts about them, and those thoughts cause feelings and behaviors. After you have a sense of what events cause negative emotions and behaviors, the next step is to identify the problematic thoughts you have about those events.

Some thoughts are known as hot thoughts because they carry emotion and are strongly connected to intense feeling. We have some thoughts which are simply about the world and are basic facts or judgments. However, some other thoughts evoke an intense feeling. Hot thoughts can be things like, "My father never appreciates what I do for him" or "I always screw up."

These thoughts are the ones you want to pay close attention to.

As you look over the situations, you've discovered that lead to problematic emotions or behaviors, think hard and evaluate what the thoughts were that lead to the emotion. For instance, maybe you became outraged when a work colleague did not reply to an email quickly. The situation was "24 hours without a reply to this email." The feeling was "anger." Maybe your behavior was "write a snarky follow-up email." What was the thought that contributed to that feeling and behavior? Perhaps it was something like "not replying to my emails is disrespecting me" or "the appropriate response to disrespect is anger."

Learning to analyze situations in the detail we have used in this chapter is crucial for being able to separate our thoughts from the situation, the feeling, and the behavior. As you learn to identify your thoughts, it can be helpful to use a daily record.

# CHAPTER 12

# REAL LIFE UTILIZATION

Congratulations! You have made it to the last step. Now, you are tasked with going out into the real world and maintaining the skills you have been developing up until this point. This is essentially you graduating from therapy.

When you go out into the real world with these skills, you will discover that you are better equipped to handling your ever-changing emotions. You will have the skills to keep yourself grounded, or at the very least, to give yourself the compassion you deserve when your anxiety symptoms do spring up again, and they will come back sometimes. Ultimately, this therapy seeks to give you the skills to manage your symptoms, so you no longer feel distressed by them, but it will never completely annihilate any feelings of anxiety. You will instead be able to recognize your anxiety as irrational and continue on with your life with that notion in mind. By disregarding your anxiety as irrational, you will feel better able to cope with the skills and not fall into the dangerous thinking traps of cognitive distortions or negative thoughts.

Try to use these skills at every opportunity that arises, as they give you control. With mindfulness, you can control your reactions to situations you have previously found troubling. Through identifying core beliefs, you will be able to identify the ways you think about yourself that are coloring your behaviors elsewhere in destructive ways. By identifying your negative thinking or cognitive distortions, you will be able to correct those as well, or at least recognize where you are likely to fall short in interacting with others. You need to recognize your weaknesses to really begin to develop your strengths, and CBT teaches you to identify your shortcomings.

Go into life knowing that CBT will not fix all of your problems, but it will teach you how to fix them. You will absolutely still feel your symptoms of anxiety sometimes. Your negative thoughts will crop up now and again and need to be re-challenged for you to regain control over them. Remember that these habits that you are trying to break are deeply ingrained in your mind and behaviors, and those behaviors will not disappear easily.

When you feel an anxiety attack coming on, use your grounding techniques and affirmations. These will help you to keep your anxiety under control. When you are able to achieve a state of mindfulness, always question your negative thoughts in order to try to challenge them so you can disregard them altogether. Remember the activities that taught you how to question your thoughts and go through the process of asking yourself if you can disprove them. When they are disproven, go through the effort of replacing your negative thought with a positive thought at the moment. Remember that an effective method of doing this is using your activity in outnumbering your negative thoughts.

Every time you have a negative thought, make it a point to replace it with something positive, or at the very least, drown it out with other positive points. Your mind will slowly adapt to using positivity when observing the world around you, and your behaviors will change to reflect this.

Now that you have a general idea of what to expect, let's consider an example. Imagine that you have social anxiety. Your friend wants you to go out to a special dinner to celebrate her promotion she has been working toward for ages at work, and after dinner, she wants you two to go out to a club for a few drinks. You happily agree, wanting to support your friend and show how happy you are for her, even though you know that you hate going out to events and social settings like those.

As the date creeps closer, you feel your anxiety coming up. Before, you would usually allow your anxiety to tell you that something bad must be coming simply by virtue of feeling anxious, but you remind yourself that that is a cognitive distortion, and you cannot use emotional reasoning to dissuade yourself to go out and support your friend. You take a few deep breaths and remind yourself of your affirmation: "I am in control of my anxiety, and even though I may feel as though I am in danger, I recognize that it is my anxiety trying to fool me." Repeating that to yourself a few times, you feel your heart rate steady, and you continue about your day.

Despite telling yourself to pay your anxiety no mind, you feel a little more tense than normal as you go about your day. At work, one of your coworkers' pokes fun at a tiny mistake you made, not meaning to insult you but to playfully tease you for a quick laugh from the two of you. Usually, you would play along, but you immediately feel your blood pressure spikes, and your anxiety starts going crazy. You can feel a strong reaction to your coworker coming, and immediately, you try to focus on your grounding techniques to steady yourself. You go through identifying things around you with your various senses, and by the time you get to the third step in the sequence, you already feel yourself calming down. You quickly ask yourself what is upsetting you, and you realize that the answer is that your coworker teased you, and as you recently learned through your activities in this book, you have an inferiority complex, and the idea of making mistakes is a huge trigger for you. Immediately, you had felt attacked and vulnerable upon hearing your coworker teasing you.

By recognizing this, you are able to appeal to the rational side of your brain, reminding yourself that it had been a joke that was not meant to offend, and you repeat yet another affirmation. "I am capable, and I am worthy of the same compassion and understanding as everyone else. Everyone makes mistakes, and that is okay." Your anxiety attack is defused before it was ever able to explode in your face, and you are feeling pretty good about yourself, as so far, you have managed to cope with your anxiety, even when it threatened to overwhelm you.

Usually, by this point in the day, you would have given in to your anxiety and felt so worked up that you would have canceled your date with your friend. Instead, using your coping skills as necessary, you have been able to manage your anxiety. Things are looking up for you, and you head home from work to get ready to meet your friend for the night.

You go home and pull out your favorite outfit for a nice night on the town. You put in on, and as you do, you realize that the top is a bit tighter than normal, and immediately put yourself down, telling yourself that you should not be eating so much, or at the very least, you should be exercising more to keep your weight in check. After telling yourself this, you realize that you had a negative thought about yourself, insulting yourself for gaining weight. Taking a deep breath, you remind yourself of three things about your appearance that you do like in order to drown out the one negative thing you said.

Feeling pretty good overall at this point, you head out to meet your friend at the restaurant. You get in and the two of you are settled in. You find that you and your friend are at a center table in the room, and again, you feel the familiar tendrils of anxiety reaching around your mind. You **hate** the inner table because of your anxiety, and it always makes you feel as though everyone is staring at you from all sides. Again, you return to your grounding techniques and take a few deep breaths. With a quiet reminder to yourself to calm down, you are able to continue throughout the night. You repeat another affirmation you use when you are feeling as though you are being watched or judged. "I am secure with who I am, and people around me likely are too busy paying attention to what they are doing to notice me."

Again, you appeal to the rational part of your mind, and you feel your anxiety flare starting to fade away. You are able to enjoy your dinner with your friend with only a few more deep breaths and affirmations when you felt your anxiety threatening to boil over again.

By the end of dinner, you are still feeling pretty in control of your emotions, although the anxiety is there, and you are aware of it. It becomes a minor annoyance that you are eventually able to tune out. You and your friend go to the club, and that is where you know your anxiety will really be tested.

The crowd, the loud noises, and the enclosed space surrounded by strangers are immediate triggers for you, and again, you must struggle to wrestle with your anxiety to remind yourself that you are in control and safe. Despite the anxiety screaming at you that something bad is going to happen, you remind yourself that your anxiety is attempting to predict the future, or a worst-case scenario and the likelihood of something bad happening there while you are enjoying your friend is slim to none. At worst, one of you might spill a drink or something.

Once again keeping your anxiety at bay, you are able to enjoy your night. The entire night was enjoyed, and while you had some close calls that definitely would have stopped you from enjoying your day before, thanks to the CBT process, you were able to keep your anxiety under control. Your friend genuinely thanks you for the experience and tells you how proud she is that you managed to get through the whole night when crowds and public events are so difficult for you.

At that moment, you feel your first major victory: You were able to get through the entire day without letting anxiety control you. Your anxiety did not cause you to back out from your time with your friend, nor did cause you to blow up at your coworker. Through the steps provided in the book and with a better understanding of how your own mind works, you were able to avoid any major mishaps engaging in one of your biggest triggers.

No matter what your individual scenario is or how it plays out, remember to use your skills in real time. Celebrate every success, no matter how small, and remember to treat yourself compassionately if you make mistakes. You are deserving of that compassion and understanding. This is not an easy process, nor is it a smooth one. You are bound to have slip-ups or mistakes, and that does not mean you are failing the process.

Before you go out on your own, here are three more skills to add to your arsenal and take with you as you attempt to navigate your triggers in real time.

# CONCLUSION

The next step is to delve into the world of self-love and self-care. You know that you need help to keep moving forward in the right direction. Otherwise, you would not have bought this book! Cognitive Behavioral Therapy is the most cutting-edge system of therapy available. It is, arguably, also the most effective. There is a reason why it has taken the United States by storm and earned its place as a top treatment plan for most psychologists today.

In fact, here are some great statistics about Cognitive Behavioral Therapy just to remind you of what a great system it is:

- It has been found CBT can be upwards of 75% effective as a single system.

- After about 8-15 sessions, 50-85% of those using it to battle anxiety and/or depression felt their symptoms were under control.

- Combining both chemical treatment (medication) and Cognitive Behavioral Therapy is the single most effective treatment method for long-term psychological disturbances.

Cognitive Behavioral Therapy is only half of the battle,

however. You must also find it within yourself, to be honest with yourself and change your entire way of thinking. Cognitive Behavioral Therapy is hard- it is not an easy path to go down. You will find endless challenges as you put all of the tenants of this treatment plan into action. The point of it is to fight through and come out swinging.

Do not be discouraged at your first relapse. No matter what, you are worthy, and you will be okay. Relapse is, inevitably, a part of recovery. You have not failed just because you were not able to complete the steps in the allotted time. You may need just to take a step back and reframe how you are thinking about the process.

It is so incredibly easy to integrate into every day. You will be so much better off for it, too.

I would recommend that the first thing you do after reading this book is to invest in either a great workbook for Cognitive Behavioral Therapy or at least a blank journal. Even just keeping track of your moods can make all the difference. Even if that is the only lesson you take away from reading my book, I will be happy! Of course, it would also be nice if you began to think about your cognitive distortions. And if you put all of the exercises into practice. I know that some of them feel a little ingenuine or even "cheesy," but I promise that they will absolutely change your life.

You deserve to live a life of freedom and relaxation. You deserve consistent, strong relationships which you feel confident in. You deserve to feel like you are the one in the driver's seat. You deserve a great night of rest, easy interpersonal relationships, and to love the person you see in the mirror. Whether you read this as a way to help you fall asleep due to insomnia or to help you bring your panic attacks under control, there is a method in this book that will solve your problem.

The only thing left to do is, well, to just do it!

CPSIA information can be obtained
at www.ICGtesting.com
Printed in the USA
BVHW041607101220
595274BV00025B/1425

9 781801 326018